THE JOCK DOC'S BODY REPAIR KIT

THE JOCK DOC'S

BODY REPAIR KIT

The New Sports Medicine for Recovery and Increased Performance

Andrew Feldman, M. D.

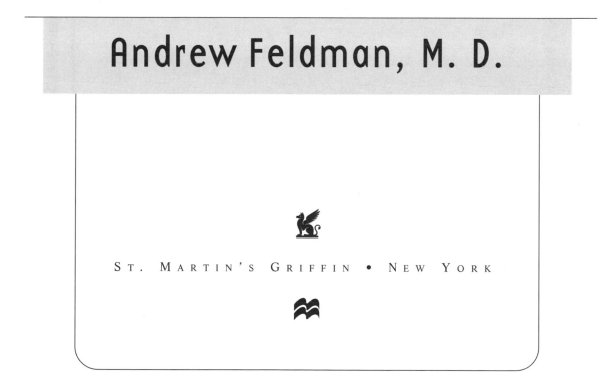

St. Martin's Griffin • New York

DEC 11 '99

DISCLAIMER: This book is not in any way intended to be the equivalent of four years of medical school and years of orthopedic training. It is instead a compendium of knowledge in the art of self-diagnosis and treatment. If at any time you feel unsure of the process or if you don't seem comfortable with your injury or the time frame it takes to improve, see a doctor.

Production Editor: David Stanford Burr

Book Design: James Sinclair

Illustrations: Precision Graphics

Library of Congress Cataloging-in-Publication Data

Feldman, Andrew.
    The jock doc's body repair kit / by Andrew Feldman.—1st
St. Martin's Griffin ed.
        p.   cm.
    ISBN 0-312-19905-8
    1. Sports medicine—Popular works. 2. Sports injuries—Prevention.
I. Title.
RC1210.F36   1999
617.1'027—dc21   98–42071
                                                        CIP

10 9 8 7 6 5 4 3 2

Acknowledgments

When I sat down to write these acknowledgments I began to ponder. Do I thank only those who have helped get the book on the shelves, or do I delve deeper to include those individuals who helped me become the person who I am; those who laid the fertile soil during my growth and allowed me to feel comfortable with myself and my accomplishments.

With this in mind, there are two specific lists of people who must be thanked. First and foremost, Eli Gottlieb, whose wit and humor is laced throughout this tome. He wears his craft like a beautiful crown, and I love him dearly. I owe a debt of gratitude to the great people at St. Martin's Press, especially Becky Koh. She "got it" when no one else did, and her guidance kept the engine running when the gas tank was on empty. Thanks also to John Murphy (the Cat's P.J.s), Sally Richardson (you can drive my car anytime), and Henry Yee for their help. Also playing a key role was my agent, Sterling Lord, who believed in the project from the start. Colleagues who, along the way, helped me through the tortures of modern medical training, were Dave Mohler at Cornell University Medical College (those late-night margaritas did truly help us become better doctors), my friend and partner Dr. Steven Sheskier—a brilliant surgeon who has kept me laughing all these years, Dr. Freddy Fu (my Zen Master), and Dr. Jim Bradley, who always lent a shoulder and sage advice. Most important, my brother-in-law, Dr. Steven Sergay, who has, and will always be, my role model. Thanks also to my residents and fellows, who have made my job that much more interesting.

The second list of people are those who have greatly influenced me over the years; those who taught me right from wrong. I owe a special thanks to my best friends, Joshua Wesson (the best heart God ever made), Paul Mones (a mo and a head), John Kilik (you will always be my roomie), and Abe Gorelick (hey Yabe). These four guys are my conscience, and I am the luckiest of men to have them as my friends. Also, Thomas Drazin, blood brother and traveling buddy.

Special, special thanks to Monika Chiang (aka The Bomb), Danny O'Neill, Peter Howes, Charlie Hebstreith, Peter Tunny, Peter Beard, Steven Warshaw (Shecky—who got the book out there), Matt Dillon, Barry Kucker, Rebel and Donna Kessler, Laura Dean, Brian Collins, Ronnie Gesser, Ty Kestner, Karen Allen, Jerry Lefcourt, Nick Parotta, Nicky and David Rabin, Lance Stern, Kathleen Turner, Brian Steele, Richard Zimmerman, Burt and Marlene Josephs, Lori Loughlin, Marty Jaramello, Dennis Fabian, Fisher Stevens, Joey "Pants," Julia Anderson, Steve Stern, Scott Stackman, Ray Quinn, Terry Quinn, Mark and Joanna Fleisher, Adam Katz, Leonie Degroot, Bruce Frankle, Paul Theophanis, Marie Medrano, Joy Medrano, Gino Medrano, Victoria Council, Karin Fossum, and David Zatzkis.

Certainly my family gets the biggest and best thanks. Milton, Ruth, Betty, Janie, Mark, Steven, Erica, Jennifer, Amanda, Samantha, Rebecca, and all Drazins and Feldmans in the New York Metropolitan area. I love you all dearly, what more can I say.

—Andrew Feldman, M.D.

Contents

THE JOCK DOC'S BODY REPAIR KIT

Introduction

There's a story I often tell patients. Once upon a time there was a man named Mr. Hasty. Mr. Hasty was a nice guy, a clean-living family man who gave at the office and at home. One afternoon on the tennis court, Mr. Hasty decided to let it all hang out. Mr. Hasty was forty, you see, and sustained the charming vanity that his body, which was reasonably fit and trim, would serve him with the same gusto it did twenty years earlier, when he was the rocket of the court. Mr. Hasty hit the ball to his business partner as if he meant to murder it. He was charged with endorphins and feeling no pain. Mr. Hasty made a booming alpha male serve that nicked the line at nearly a hundred per—and then fell down clutching his knee and howling like a wounded animal.

Delusions of youth strike again!

As an orthopedic surgeon, one of the chief things I see in my practice is the athletic equivalent of cognitive dissonance—people, who for reasons of ego or ignorance, misjudge the capabilities of their bodies to perform and order them to extremes that damage them, painfully, and often expensively, too. As in the sad case of Mr. Hasty, much of the problem comes from the ghost of athletics past. On the one hand, enormous strides have been made in prolonging the capacities of bones and muscles to retain their elasticity for far longer than ever before. But people take this as a kind of license to get up and let it rip. They see someone on TV competing in Masters bicycling or swimming or lacrosse, and they leap from their BarcaLoungers in great sprays of potato chips and say "I can do that too!" The sad truth is, you can as soon perform a tonsillectomy with a Bic pen.

The body is a fabulously complicated and wonderful machine—the result of millions of years of evolution. The more I've learned about it, the more amazed I've become at its seamless precision and efficiency. Its healing powers are astonishing. It is able to effortlessly regenerate broken bones, grow flesh and nerves across shattered gaps, meld torn ligaments together. Its brain and organs can adapt to a staggering amount of toxins and disabilities and still function. The natural healing response of the body is one of its more powerful and basic impulses, and doctors, despite their often knowing air, are in reality only playing follow the leader. The body dictates. The body, to adapt a more contemporary parlance, rules. And yet, as wonderfully complex and powerful as it is, the body has its very specific limits, and though those limits can be extended through careful training and diet, one cannot simply take a header into the fountain of youth at whim. I know quite well about the injuries sustained through the sudden decision to rashly, and without preparation, launch oneself into sports. How do I know, you may ask? Because of my experiences with—what else—*my* body.

MY BODY

Here's what I've done to it in a career of manic amateur athleticism: torn the ligaments in my left ankle three times; broken three fingers and my nose twice (once playing basketball and once, I'm afraid, lifting weights); separated my shoulder and tore the ligament in my left thumb while skiing; suffered a healthy baker's dozen from tendonitis and bursitis; and have endured intermittent lower back pain since age eighteen.

I was a hyperactive child in the balmy pre-Ritalin days when the only therapy for kids like me was sports: the therapy "worked," because to this day I am obsessed with sports. I work out at least once in the evening, and follow it up whenever possible with a chaser of tennis, basketball, skiing, or touch football in the park. My point in this recitation is that I know it from both sides of the fence. I've been there—banged, bruised, and upset—in the doctor's office, and I've also been the guy in the white coat, making the diagnosis, holding the knife.

Perhaps it was this two-track experience that allowed me, once I became a doctor, to understand a small but important fact: *90 percent of all sports medical injuries are the same.* They have exactly the same damage patterns and the same recovery rates. This is not exactly earth-shattering news, but it tends to be overlooked by the weekend warriors streaming into my office with worried looks on their faces. The fact bears repeating: 90 percent of sports medical injuries are the same. And really, why shouldn't they be? Despite the claims of certain politicians, we are all, from a medical standpoint, more or less identical. Just as sports themselves are performed according to specific and very uniform rules, the injuries, too, tend to occur in very specific and predictable ways: The same torque (twist) will produce the same tear, no matter what game is being played.

I was drawn to the idea of writing this book because it occurred to me that, with a little of the right information, many of my patients could have spared themselves the expense and time of a medical visit. What was needed, it seemed to me, was a book that contained all the useful medical facts, but without the off-putting jargon; a book that allowed you to perform a simple at-home diagnostic exam for each pain or injured body part, and empowered YOU to make the determination whether or not to see the doctor. This last point can't be stressed too much. Injuries tend to render us passive, dependent, and in the worst cases, hopeless. Part of the reason for this is simple lack of information. Fear—often a side effect of ignorance—is a huge negative motivator, both on the playing fields and off. This book will help vanquish the dark fearful clouds that so often accompany sports injuries. The body, except in the rare cases of catastrophic injury, will heal itself quickly and efficiently, and with the help of this book and your own healing response, you'll soon be back in the game.

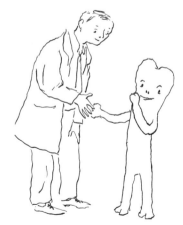

To assist us in this enterprise, I'd like to introduce my slightly unwilling protégé and addled assistant, Bone Boy. He'll be along for the journey and, when he's not being cranky, is actually a nice guy. Bone Boy, will you take a bow please?

"Stick with me, boys and girls, I'll tell you all you need to know."

MY AIM

My aim in the pages that follow is to take the pomposity out of the white coat and to impart my knowledge of fifteen years of medical training into something that is user-friendly and useful to boot. Part of that has meant providing some in-flight entertainment along the way. These are included not only to make you smile. I believe that the personal touch is what counts in medicine, and I want you to know—and trust—me entirely. In addition to slices of "My Own Private Idaho," there is the medical meat of this book: an overview of each body part, an understanding of its anatomical function, a history of its injury patterns, and specific directions on how best to diagnose the extent of the damage, and most speedily remedy it. This self-diagnostic process, gathered together in what I call the *Bio-Point Exam*, will allow you to proceed along a series of simple yes/no questions until you figure out what's wrong, and then direct you to the appropriate therapy.

For those light moments in which you simply want a guided tour of that most fascinating of theme parks, the human body, or those more serious times when the twinge has already taken place, the ankle has been twisted, the gremlins of aches and pains have lodged in that overused knee or shoulder or elbow, *Jock Doc* will give you the words and techniques to take control of the situation and put you at your ease. Think of the book as a twenty-four-hour roadside assistance program for your body, which will keep you running smooth and clean on the highway of improved sports performance.

Part One

The Doctor Is In

1

Injuries, Diagnosis, and Treatment

INJURIES

My nephew Alan describes the scene: He is sitting doing his homework in the living room one evening when his fifty-something father Dave comes bounding up the stairs, belly floating zeppelinlike out over his pants, and stands there waving his arms and trash-talking like Larry Bird. "My sky-hook was jammin', honey!" he shouts to his wife. "I just nailed the game-winner, now gimme a kiss!"

No, my nephew is not delusional. This really happened. And, in fact, the scene of formerly housebound moms and dads becoming competitive athletes at a time of life previously reserved for high-impact bridge and needlepoint is now being repeated en masse all over the country. From senior baseball leagues, to the senior circuit in tennis and golf, and the Master's Olympics, the "calendrically challenged" are rising up and hitting the courts harder and in greater numbers than ever before.

Of course, twenty-year-olds get injured too, as do thirty-year-olds for that matter. And they get injured in greater numbers and in more bizarre ways than ever before. The advent of rollerblading, windsurfing, snow- and skateboarding, and other nouveau sports whose operative words are: "let it rip, dude!" tend to provoke serious injury rates with entirely new injury patterns.

Chronic Versus Acute Injuries

The recent demographic earthquake in sports has brought with it some serious medical consequences. One of the most pronounced is the rise in *repetitive use* or *overuse injuries*. Although the resultant pain of overuse or chronic injuries versus that of acute injuries is vaguely similar, and the joint afflicted may be the same one, medically speaking they occupy different universes. An *acute injury* is one in which the anatomy of the limb or joint was changed dramatically, usually by a trauma. *Chronic injuries* are the result of day-in-day-out microtraumatic responses that slowly add up over time, and finally render the limb symptomatic. These injuries are usually the result of small imperfections in the type or quantity of movements you make when exercising, added to whatever various structural defects exist in your body. They are tricky to prevent, because there's no dramatic smashup—no blaze of powder snow and snapping ski poles; no sudden, sickening crash into the Zamboni at the ice-skating rink. Rather than obvious, they are insidious, silent, and destructive (like compound interest).

Your golf grip is wrong; your butterfly stroke is erratically executed; your jogging stride is off—any of these fairly innocent things, multiplied by a million repetitions, can add up to walloping aches and pains. Take tennis elbow, the bane of amateur players the world over. The prevailing myth is that tennis elbow is simply the result of playing too much—and like most myths, there's a kernel of truth in it. But often there are complicating factors having to do with a wrong grip, a racket strung at the incorrect tension for you, or improper form.

A Thought About Form

I have no desire to rain cold medical facts on anyone's parade, but the truth is that in certain situations, not even the most perfect prize-winning form in the world will save you from injury. Given today's political climate, I might be accused of "bodism" in saying this, but I must: some bodies are simply not cut out for particular sports—and not all the titanium accessories or high-priced personal trainers will change the fact. Certain examples come to mind. Persons afflicted with very flat feet should stay away from running marathons because the shock of those millions of footsteps will be transmitted directly to their knees and hips and cause a world of trouble. If you have "knock knees" (the medical term is valgus), you shouldn't be pounding the pavement at length either. Scoliosis or curvature of the spine? Eliminate all attempts at the Tour de France—the stresses involved in positioning yourself atop a bicycle for even modest recreational trips will cause the agony jet to begin to roar.

As a doctor, it is sometimes quite difficult for me to explain to my hopeful patients that a favorite activity is off-limits for the sake of their health, but as a responsible practitioner, I have no choice. Orthotics and braces can sometimes help to correct certain weaknesses (see Chapter 10), but in specific cases, the wiser choice is simply to change one's sport. The moral of the story? Better to retain your health and narrow the scope of your athletic activities than remain heroically versatile—and bedridden.

Patience Is a Sporting Virtue

Often, overuse injury is the result not of bad form or structural defect, but of rushing too far too fast. The importance of a training program is precisely that it gives the body those critical intervals to recover and regenerate. I'm always telling marathoners-in-training to slow down their intervals, to work in gradual phases and follow a routine that allows them to progress by degrees, rather than through an explosive jump forward. For those who have already injured a body part but require the aerobic pump of sustained exertion, I usually advise cross-training. This gives the cardiovascular workout that's needed while distributing the pressure of athletic activity around the body. And a good cross-training routine can be tailored to your individual needs. Sore shoulder keeping you off the tennis court? Nip this pretendonitis in the bud by trying a step aerobics class or possibly a rowing machine until the twinge passes. Your knee feeling like it can't take another flight of stairs? Head for the swimming pool. Before you do anything, however, you should make absolutely certain you work out a deep, searching, and disciplined routine of stretching.

The Joy of Stretch

No matter the sport, no matter the body type or character, there is a key piece of advice I dole out regularly to all recreational athletes: that advice is to stretch! I know, I know: it's harder than it sounds. Cold muscles are not especially friendly creatures, and besides, stretching takes up a serious chunk of time. Many is the time I've driven to a nearby jogging track and found, as I arrive, that the clouds have parted, the track is deserted, and sun is pouring down. The scene is picture-perfect, and the question is obvious: Why spend twenty minutes on the infield twisted like a Bachman's pretzel when I can get right out on the track and watch the cinders fly?

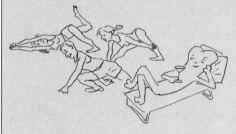

"I love stretching, I could watch it all day!"

Stretching is not glamorous; nor is it especially satisfying to the endorphin-addicted. It is merely the best, most time-tested way of boosting athletic performance and ensuring the longevity of muscles that has ever been discovered. Stretching lengthens the muscles and lubricates the joints, preparing them for athletic endeavor; and, by warming muscle fibers, it speeds contraction rate and oxygen efficiency. It gently prods the heart to a gallop, rather than kickstarting it explosively. As you grow older, your cartilaginous tissues and tendons shrink like the rubber parts of a car left in the sun—they have decreased blood flow and an increased tendency to become stiff and arthritic. The older you are, the more important it is that you warm up your muscles. Not only will you play better, and gain a competitive edge, your chance of injury will nosedive.

Never ever—and especially after age forty—should you go directly from your street clothes to tennis togs and booming serves. It may be helpful if you actually think of stretching as *part of the game*, a fifteen to forty minute interlude, which should be factored into all your plans and schedules. As to the stretching routine itself, remember: the body is pure interactivity, and every muscle system participates in nearly every physical action. Your stretching, therefore, should aim at a generalized routine, which includes all muscles, and not merely those being most heavily stressed in the sport to follow. For example, if you jog, you should also do a shoulder workout. If you swim, be sure to stretch the Achilles tendon.

If you need inspiration to keep you stretching, look no further than professional sports—specifically, the pitcher in the bull pen. When the pitcher on the mound begins to throw wild, the relief pitcher in the bull pen gets to work. Watch him carefully, because he always follows the same routine. First, he does some simple stretches, often with the help of a trainer. Then he throws some light tosses. Then he begins a slow velocity windup, and only then, when his body is fully warmed and stretched, does he begin throwing with real heat. Pitchers, remember, are professional athletes, who do this every day, are in peak physical condition, and have probably already stretched that morning. They follow this routine of stretching and warm-up for a very simple reason: *they want their arms to last*.

Appendix B, Rehab Exercises and Stretches, will show you exactly what stretching you should do. NBA star Kareem Abdul Jabbar attributed his phenomenal longevity as a player to his yoga-inspired regiment of stretching. Ladies and Gentlemen, stretch!

DIAGNOSIS

Let's talk about diagnosis. Diagnosis is the beginning of the treatment process for an incoming patient. It also happens to be one of my favorite aspects of medicine. Diagnosis is an adventure of intellect and education, a sleuthing of a sort in which the doctor, as a kind of forensic Colombo, minus the filthy London Fog and smelly cigar, walks into a room and tries to solve the case of the injury. What were you doing when it happened? What have you tried to remedy it? Has the injury ever gone away and then returned, or has it been a progressive problem? Those, and a dozen other questions are the typical beginning of my interview with a patient. I look at his or her posture and body alignment. I observe his or her general state of muscle tone. I attempt to find out if unconscious repetitive movements in his or her job or at home may have contributed to the condition. After the questions and answers, I do a physical exam, gently flexing and torquing the area around the injury. Depending on the severity of the injury, X rays may be necessary. When all is said and done, I take the clues and try to solve the crime. It is precisely this problem-solving sequence that this book will place in your hands.

I should mention that the state of diagnostic medicine is considerably different from what it was—even fifteen years ago. This is so for a very good reason: medical science never sleeps—literally. In an effort to mimic and better understand what happens when you run, walk, or stretch to rifle a crosscourt tennis shot back over the net, machines work all night long in the basements of labs the world over. Cadaver ligaments attached to strain gauges on machines that resemble bicycles are endlessly repeating small motions in an effort to find the weak point. In what was until recently merely a Frankenstein-flavored fantasy, researchers are working on growing replacement cell cartilage and bionic joints in laboratories, and the outcomes of patients in large control groups are being closely monitored and factored. Inspired by magnetic resonance imaging (MRI), technicians are in a race to find the next best radiological diagnostic tools. Why is all this necessary? Because regardless of how sophisticated and efficient we become, there will always be injuries.

TREATMENT

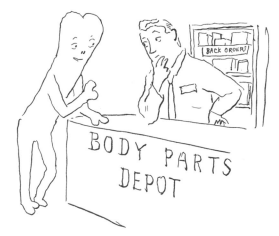

"Yes, I'd like George Clooney's haircut and Matt Dillon's cheekbones, please."

Before I get into the anatomical specifics, I'd like to sketch for you my philosophy on treating injuries so that you know what you'll be dealing with in forthcoming chapters. Basically, I'd describe it as Realistic, writ large. I have been trained, over about a billion hours, in a very specific type of classical Western medicine. And yet if one thing is clear to me, it's that no one, not even the mighty colossus of Modern Medicine, has a monopoly on the biological truth. My point? That if you feel like it, you're welcome to try alternatives. That's right: an orthopedic surgeon without any alcohol in his bloodstream is telling you that you might actually get something out of yoga, massage, meditation, or acupuncture. As long as it's noninvasive and doesn't hurt you, my attitude is: why not? The science of healing is full of twists and turns and medical surprises. I could—but won't—begin a long discussion on the restorative powers of laughter, sunshine, and that vague but important elixir, "the will to live." There are specialists who believe that sitting inside a hyperbaric chamber like a herring in a tin can makes you heal faster, and there are devotees of yoga who regularly run a length of gauze through their nose and mouth and then tug it back and forth to clean the sinuses. The bottom line? Don't go crazy, but keep an open mind.

When it comes to the treatment itself, my credo is, less is more. I will treat a patient by any means necessary, but conservative treatment is the time-tested best. Our bodies are supremely adaptable, and come to us preprogrammed with the knowledge of how best to heal. Most of the time, in the case of injuries, the wisest course is to encourage that healing process through noninvasive means, such as bracing, physical therapy, and acupuncture, rather than jumping scalpel-first into the driver's seat. The usual first step in any treatment process, when indicated, is RICE, which stands for rest, ice, compression, and elevation. In addition, stretching or physical therapy, possibly a cortisone injection or a change in footwear may be called for. For repetitive or overuse injuries, judicious use of anti-inflammatory medicine is often helpful. Let me repeat the word, *judicious*. You may substitute the word controlled, or moderate. Too often people assume that if a medication is sold over the counter, it can be taken at double or triple the recommended dose, and function three times as effectively. This is simply not true. All medications carry side effects with them, and the chronic abuse of anti-inflammatories, for example, can lead to decidedly unglamourous holes in the stomach and even more severe problems.

With musculoskeletal injuries—in distinction to life generally—time is usually your best friend. On the other hand, with certain injuries, such as bone spurs, all the time in the world won't help heal you. As a last resort, if medication, rest, stretching, and other avenues have been fully explored, then and only then will surgery be used.

SURGERY

I cut people for a living: I take the knife or the basket forceps in the knee, shave the cartilage smooth, insert the gleaming titanium parts of a joint replacement. But this only happens in a very small percentage of my cases. How small? Would you believe about 10 percent? As the saying goes, "There is nothing wrong that surgery can't make worse."

Mind you, the word "surgery" has an entirely different meaning today from its meaning thirty years ago, say, when knee surgery, for example, was an expensive, painful, and time-consuming operation, with a high risk of infection, which often had the patient laid up in bed for weeks. The arthroscope has revolutionized orthopedic surgery as we know it, and many procedures today are no more invasive than going to the dentist to have your teeth drilled. A side result of "Surgery Lite" is that medicine has inadvertently become the designer field of the '90s. If you don't have your own personal sports medicine doctor and at least two or three suture holes on your knee, you're going to be laughed right out of certain cocktail parties. Arthroscopic procedures are so common these days that I often (at these same parties) hear people rating their doctors on speed, comfort, and finesse at hiding scars, in the same way that people used to talk about their cars or horses.

And now that you've chosen the right surgeon, let us talk about the place he or she spends most of his or her time concentrating on: the body.

One of the common misconceptions about the arthroscope is that it is a kind of magic wand, a super-healer that can correct everything from tonsillitis to male-pattern baldness. Patients come to me regularly, saying, "Can you scope my tendonitis and fix it, Doc?" The answer, I'm afraid, is no, for a simple reason: the arthroscope can treat certain kinds of injuries involving joints, ligaments, and tendons—but not all of them.

Is all this surgery necessary? Yes, and no. For acute, traumatic events (Yes, Virginia, bad things do happen to good bodies) such as tears in the ligaments, tendons, or cartilage, surgery is often the only option. But with the more chronic injuries such as tendonitis or bursitis, conservative treatment is more often the method of choice.

Choosing a Doctor

Given the upheaval in medical practice and insurance, there is a better than even chance that you'll change doctors somewhere down the line, and that you'll experience that anxiety-producing moment in which you meet an unknown person who will soon be handling, treating, or possibly even cutting into a sensitive body part. How to make this experience less nerve-racking? Here are some points I recommend you bear in mind.

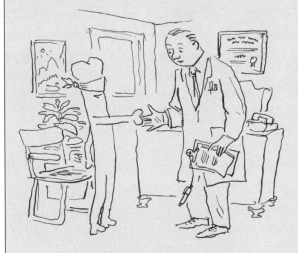

"So glad to meet you Doctor, you look like just the man for the job."

Manner, first. A good doctor is an open doctor, a doctor who puts you at your ease, who gives you the experience of being listened to and talked to on an equal level. You should feel comfortable and the atmosphere should be both candid and pleasant. There is no illness or discomfort so standard that a patient's input about it is not valuable. Has the doctor solicited your story from you? Has he or she listened in detail? Surgery is a technical art, and surgeons must not only have good motor skills, but clean and orderly thought patterns. Do the doctor's explanations in response to your questions satisfy your desire to know? There is nothing wrong with asking as many questions as you feel necessary or with soliciting a second opinion, and a good doctor will not be defensive when you bring up the possibility of doing so.

Which brings me to references, a word that works on two levels. On the one hand, there are social references—people who you meet at the gym, while jogging, or at cocktail parties, who speak glowingly of a certain doctor. (If you're in doubt about who to ask, just look for the person with the brace; physical therapists at gyms are also good bets.) These kinds of references, especially if plentiful about a particular doctor, generally tend to indicate a good bet. If you are contemplating seeing a particular surgeon, don't be shy about asking around about him or her. Ask your GP or internist, if you have one, as he or she may have have information that can be useful. But you are also entirely within your rights, if you feel a bit confused or doubtful, *to solicit patient references from a doctor*. In my own practice I often find that patients, especially when fearful about an operation, take great comfort from talking to a patient who has undergone the same procedure.

Attendance at a top medical school is no guarantee of a good doctor, but I, for one, would rather see a diploma from an A-list institution on the wall of my surgeon's office than one from the Bakelite College of Medicine. On a related note, don't be afraid to ask the doctor if he or she has had fellowship training, which is additional training in a specialty that is undertaken after completing a four or five year medical residency program.

Ask if the doctor has performed this procedure often, and listen carefully to his explanation of the surgery itself. The explanations should include alternative treatment methods, if possible. The doctor should be very, very clear. Whether he uses verbal, visual, or even acoustic aids, he should explain EXACTLY what he's going to do, and why. Doctors who present their case for surgery in clean, precise terms, usually tend to perform the surgery itself in similar fashion.

This is the Information Age, and there is an avalanche of data available to the public about all surgical procedures. The only downside of this is that occasionally patients become overly stuffed with information and feel themselves whipsawed by competing opinions and outlooks. The world of medicine is phenomenally complex and intricate, which is why the irrefutable fact of a doctor you can trust is of such primary importance. Trust—its establishment, care, and feeding—is the most important bond between a surgeon and patient. You'll know your orthopedic surgeon anywhere from two months to over a year. Establishing trust at the outset is the fastest way of reducing anxiety about the entire process.

Part Two

The Body Shop

WELCOME TO MY OFFICE

Generally speaking, people with athletic injuries tend to have localized problems. As opposed to infection, which can make your entire body feel like The Great Dismal Swamp, sports injuries are tidily specific, and usually afflict individual joints or limbs. I say this by way of introduction to the beating heart of this book: the following chapters deal with the injuries themselves. For ease of access, I've keyed all the diagnostics in the ensuing chapters to their respective body parts. Find the chapter pertinent to your problem, and start from there. Each chapter contains an overview of the limb and its physical function, and some anatomical background, too. The anatomy is important both to give you a mental picture of the injury site, and to allow you to approach the healing process with the calm that comes from being informed. Along with anatomy is background on typical injuries and some typical treatments—all of which is designed to help put you in the driver's seat of your own rehabilitation. Once you've digested these sections, the first place you'll drive to is that little self-diagnostic marvel called the Bio-Point Exam.

SELF-DIAGNOSIS AND YOU

People these days are increasingly grabbing the reins of their own lives, directing matters to improve their health and well-being. They do this for the best of reasons—they want to prolong and maximize their physical performance in life. But they do it also, I think, because they're skeptical about what they see going on in the world around them. People these days are skeptical about *everything*—the nightly news; the promises of politicians; myths of progress; the salaries of athletes and actors; they're skeptical—increasingly—about doctors, too. Who to trust in these corrosive times? I have a simple answer: trust your body. It's not trying to sell you anything. It has no angle. It needs only to be listened to on its own terms, and it will dependably reward you for you investment of time and attention.

If that doesn't convince you to take self-diagnosis seriously, think about this: as a result of the recent trend toward breast self-examination, women's mortality rate from breast cancer has fallen by 25 percent over the last twenty years. Are you a believer yet? I hope so.

The Bio-Point Exams designed for each body part will allow you to take an active role in your own diagnosis and treatment. By answering simple yes/no questions, you will proceed along a ladder of possibilities until you figure out what your injury is, and if it requires you to see a doctor. The Bio-Point Exam has been designed to provide you with the most focused, efficient, at-home diagnosis currently available. The Bio-Point Exam procedure consists of two parts. In the first part, you will determine the severity of your injury by answering a series of five very basic questions. This will allow you to decide whether or not you qualify for self-treatment or must see a doctor. Having cleared this first section, you will proceed to Part Two, where you will be led through a self-exam, which will zero in on your muscular-skeletal problem, diagnose them, and then supply the appropriate treatment and exercises to rehabilitate the injury.

There is no rush. It is not a tax audit and there are no right or wrong answers. There is only accuracy—it is important that your answers reflect the truth as far as you know it. If self-treatment is indicated, you will then be directed to the correct *Med-Unit* (in Appendix A), a compilation of timetables, treatments, and exercises, designed to get you back in the game as quickly as possible.

Before you begin a Bio-Point Exam, sit back a moment and try to think if your soreness, stiffness, or pain is the result of a sudden burst of athletic activity on your part. If you haven't been out on the playing courts or fields or courses for a long time, and you suddenly go out and play a sport hard—any sport—there will always be discomfort and soreness.

I speak from a vast and memorable firsthand experience in this area. There was the time I lifted weights enthusiastically after a long absence from the weight room—and had to take sponge baths and order in from the local Chinese restaurant for the next three days. There was the time I laughingly agreed to take an aerobics class with my girlfriend, explaining that I normally didn't indulge in such idle low-impact exercise—and then lay in bed the entire evening afterward like a kind of giant Klondike Bar, packed in ice.

The myth I'm trying to blow to bits for your edification is this one: that being "in shape" means being able to do anything athletic without worry. It doesn't. Being "in shape" is sports-specific, and means that your body understands the muscular and aerobic requirements for *a particular athletic activity*. You can be a bicycle sprint champ and find your leg muscles on fire after a half hour of rollerblading—and vice versa.

Point to remember: several days of soreness after sudden muscular exertion are normal, and not to worry over.

And now, onto the body in question: *yours*.

2

Shoulder

One afternoon a couple of years ago, a man came into my office. He was in his early thirties, red in the face, and obviously quite agitated. He had barely sat down in his chair when he burst into an enraged tirade against doctors. "One doctor told me I had bursitis!" he shouted. "I went to another who diagnosed tendonitis! Yet another told me I had rotator cuff syndrome! And another said inflammation of the muscles in my shoulder! Which is it, huh? You're all a bunch of crooks!"

I sat back in my chair and waited for him to quiet down. I sympathized with this poor fellow who was bewildered by what seemed to be conflicting diagnoses for his shoulder pain. I understood his confusion quite well. And when he had grown quieter, I leaned forward and explained to him the reason for his problem: all of his diagnoses meant more or less the same thing.

The shoulder joint is a miracle of design and engineering, a triumph of evolutionary adaptation. Imagine a seal balancing a ball on its nose while playing Bach on the piano and you might have an—admittedly simplistic—idea of what we're talking about. No joint is more complex than the shoulder, and none more misunderstood and misdiagnosed. Even to someone who has studied its structure, the shoulder—with its interlocking struts and sockets—still remains magical: 360 degrees of circumferential motion, an incredible arc that is unique in the body.

And yet such exquisite mechanical gifts come with a price—in this case, vulnerability. In doctor-speak, the shoulder has sacrificed stability for mobility. Able to windmill all day long, it is also easily injured. This is made worse by the sad fact that many sports, even good old-fashioned all-American apple-pie sports, rely on motions that are hostile to the shoulder. Examples? The spike in volleyball; the serve in tennis; the pitch in baseball; the drive in golf; the butterfly stroke in swimming (better, in truth, left to butterflies). When I say hostile, I mean fundamentally opposed to the future healthy functioning of that limb. Are you beginning to see the pattern? The shoulder will allow a phenomenally varied set of activities, but it has certain preferences: it doesn't exactly like being used for overhead motions. Weekend baseballers take note: this joint balks at too many overhead fastballs.

But wait, there's more!

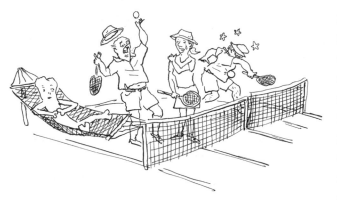

"The doctor says overhead motions are hard on the shoulder. I'm taking the news lying down."

The shoulder is, in fact, full of possibilities for mishap. "My shoulder hurts, Doc," can mean any of two dozen different things—as the red-faced man in my office found out to his chagrin. There are the fantastic variety of neck and shoulder sorenesses that accumulate in people who type too much, who drive too long, who play a sport too hard, or who just hold themselves too rigid. And then there is the roll call of the more serious medical complications: a shoulder can pop completely out of joint; a shoulder can go partially out of joint; muscles can be ripped; muscles can be inflamed; tendons can be inflamed, torn or irritated; and a host of other unpleasant possibilities.

One of the reasons we doctors see so many shoulder injuries these days among both professional and amateur athletes has to do with the emotional climate of our culture, which is fixated not only on athletic performance, but increasingly on athletic *power*. Athletes are required to move and decelerate faster than they ever were before, and the body hasn't quite gotten with the program. Let me back up a second and explain. In the 1950s, to take an example, there weren't more than a handful of pitchers who threw fastballs at 100 mph. Yet the power pitchers of today, bolstered by advances in training, medicine, and equipment now break 100 mph on a regular basis. The same thing can be said for championship tennis players. Up until recently, the hand-to-eye finesse of a "touch" player like McEnroe, was enough to land him in the winner's circle. These days it requires a 125-mph serve, shotgun ground strokes, and the stamina of a triathlete. The power game of tennis has taken over from the gentlemanly thrust and parry of once upon a time. Fine, you say. Change is great, you add. I agree. My point is only that as a culture we've become so *obsessed* with athletic performance that we've done so at a certain cost to health. Evolutionary changes take millions of years, not generations. No matter how many kinesiologists and trainers argue to the contrary, I find it hard to believe that the Creator's plans for the average shoulder included the serves of Pete Sampras.

ANATOMY

If you glance at Fig. 2.1 you'll immediately see the great reason for the shoulder's vulnerability: the head of the main arm bone is seated only shallowly in the socket of the joint. Imagine the stability of a ball sitting in a flat dish versus a ball sitting in a deep bowl, and you'll get the picture. Being only shallowly seated, the shoulder easily pops out under wrenching stress or overuse of the wrong kind.

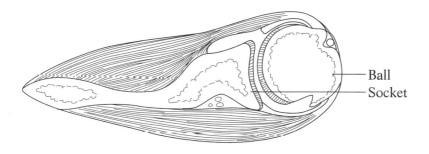

—Ball
—Socket

Fig. 2.1 Normal shoulder.

This is made even more delicate by the fact that the joint of the shoulder has no bony or skeletal sanction: there are only soft tissues keeping the shoulder together. And the ligaments of the shoulder are particularly weak. Think of that next time you throw a whizzing fastball! Bones there are aplenty in the structure of the shoulder: the clavicle, the scapula, the humerus or upper bone of the arm. But at a crucial intersection of the ball and socket, there is the infamous rotator cuff to help keep things together. Made up of four individual muscles—the supraspinatus, infraspinatus, teres minor, and subscapularis (there *will* be a quiz)—the rotator cuff forms a tight seal around the ball and socket joint. When damaged, the entire function of the shoulder is affected.

The shoulder is beloved by muscles, and has a lot of them terminating there, particularly those of the neck and torso: the deltoid, the trapezius, the pectoralis major (or "pecs" in the weight room) and the latissimus dorsi (or "lats"). They are tucked and rolled around the joint like a kind of organic upholstery, and provide the shoulder with its strength. To protect the joint itself, the shoulder is housed in something called a shoulder capsule. This is a cartilaginous bag, which holds and protects the ball and socket somewhat like the blue velvet sack does a bottle of Chivas Regal.

INJURIES

Leaving aside for a moment the many muscular and overuse-related aches and pains of the shoulder, there are two main categories of problems that often require medical attention: dislocations (along with subluxations or partial dislocation) and rotator cuff injuries.

Dislocation

Dislocation (Fig. 2.2) takes place when the head of the arm bone or humerus is wrenched completely out of the joint—à la the famous scene of the drowned guy caught in a branch in the movie *Deliverance*.

"Isn't it a shame when cousins marry?"

Often there is an actual popping sound—the body's version of a rimshot. Dislocation is usually accompanied by damage to the surrounding soft tissues and its supporting cast of nerves and blood vessels. It often, but not always, requires surgery and a period of rehabilitation, usually lasting a minimum of two months.

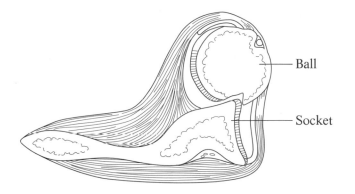

Fig. 2.2 Dislocated shoulder.

Subluxation

The lesser version of dislocation is something called subluxation, which takes place when the shoulder comes only *partially* out of the joint. A subluxer is a person who may have previously suffered a dislocation and as a result has a laxity or looseness in the joint. Where does this looseness come from? The shoulder capsule, which holds and protects the ball and socket. Once the shoulder capsule has been stretched through trauma or a repetitive-use injury, it doesn't snap back to its original size, but rather sits baggily, allowing the ball and socket more play than it should have. In these cases, it has to be hemmed surgically, somewhat like a dress.

In rare cases, subluxation can come about from a congenital problem—for example, you're born with tissues that are too stretchy.

Too what?

Yes, stretchy. Remember back in grade school, there was always a doof who would get the girls to look at him by voluntarily popping his shoulder out at a party? He had the congenital gift—or curse—of stretchy tissue.

Rotator Cuff Injuries

Everyone is familiar with this term by now, usually from reading it in a sentence about major league pitchers being placed on the disabled list (and still, I might add, collecting their multimillion dollar salaries). If dislocation and subluxation are the Harvard of shoulder injuries, then rotator cuff injuries are the Yale.

To understand rotator cuff problems you have to understand that the tendons and muscles of the body are not simply attached to the ends of bones, but are often routed through elaborate skeletal tunnels and channels on their way. A particular tunnel exists in the shoulder, where, as you raise your arm, the rotator cuff muscles slide through an opening. In doctor-talk this opening is formed by the acromion (Fig. 2.3). To my patients I often use the metaphor of the Lincoln Tunnel. Although many people are born with a normal Lincoln Tunnel, a select few are born with a Lincoln Tunnel whose aperture is too small. Thus traffic (i.e., the rotator cuff muscles) have a tough time sliding through. However, the same kind of problem can also occur in a normal shoulder when muscles swell through overuse or trauma (Fig. 2.4.). The inflammation can either resolve itself or worsen and cause ripping and tearing of the tissue.

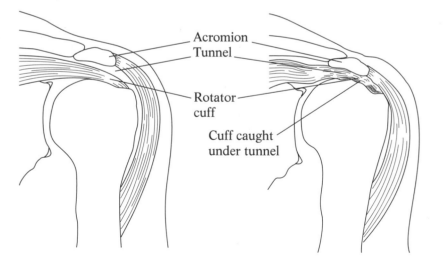

Acromion
Tunnel

Rotator cuff

Cuff caught under tunnel

Fig. 2.3 Normal rotator cuff.   **Fig. 2.4 Rotator cuff impingement.**

Other Shoulder Injuries

Did you think it ended with dislocation and subluxation? Not quite. The shoulder is cursed with a delicate fulcrum and long levers—the arms. The upshot of this is a host of happy Latinate syndromes from which the shoulder can suffer. These include **tendonitis, tenosynovitis** (inflammation of a tendon sheath), and **bursitis** (inflammation of the lubricating pouches or bursae that surround the joint). There are strains to the **trapezius** muscle, which arise mostly through tension, posture, and job-related stress, and there are the various difficulties that accrue around the **AC joint**, the big bumpy bone sitting on the top of your shoulder. It can either be separated from violent trauma (hockey players often get it from being checked into the boards), or can simply wear out from chronic inflammation. **Biceps rupture** anyone? This is another lovely shoulder-problem scenario, in which the biceps tendon literally snaps, causing a misshapen Popeye-like swelling in the arm as the freed muscle tissue retracts back up toward the shoulder. Add to this another dozen or so sprains, strains, contusions, and various arthritic conditions, and you can see that all your shoulder is asking for is a little love and respect.

Now that you have an understanding of the anatomy of the shoulder and its most common injuries, let's continue on to Part One of the Bio-Point Exam.

The BIO-POINT Exam

Shoulder

PART ONE

Question 1

Is there any deformity in the afflicted area? Look in the mirror and if possible compare the affected and the unaffected side. Is there a lack of symmetry?
If "yes," see a doctor immediately.
If "no," read on.

Question 2

Is there a severe limitation in your range of motion? Are you incapable of performing basic household tasks with the afflicted extremity?
If "yes," see a doctor immediately.
If "no," read on.

Question 3

Is there any sign of extensive or excessive swelling?
If "yes," see a doctor immediately.
If "no," read on.

Question 4

Are you afflicted with severe weakness in the injured body part? Do you have difficulty, for example, gripping a can?
If "yes," see a doctor immediately.
If "no," read on.

Question 5

Was a loud "pop" heard at the time of the injury?
If "yes," see a doctor immediately.
If "no," read on.

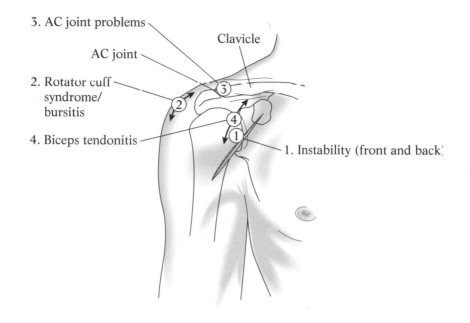

3. AC joint problems

Clavicle

AC joint

2. Rotator cuff
syndrome/
bursitis

③

②

④

①

4. Biceps tendonitis

1. Instability (front and back)

PART TWO

Whew! You're still with me! That's very good news because it means your injury may fall within the guidelines of what is treatable at home. What I'm going to do now is to zero in on your problem and attempt to make a more accurate diagnosis. Look at the accompanying illustration and touch the area where your pain or discomfort is most specific and localized. Note the number and the name of the injury (on the illustration) that corresponds with this area. Based on the area of pain you've indicated, this is likely to be the correct diagnosis. However, remember that injuries often overlap! Therefore, I recommend that you don't leap to any conclusions. Follow through by doing *all* of the Bio-Point Exams. This will ensure the most accurate and informed assessment of your injury. To help guide you in determining your own injury, each exam includes typical comments from patients suffering from that particular injury. After each exam, the page number of the corresponding Med Unit is given. The Med Units are in Appendix A. Note: If no Med Unit is given, immediate medical attention is advised—since the condition cannot be treated at home. By following the Med Unit instructions, you can begin treating your injury immediately, keeping close track of your progress as you go.

1. Instability

COMMENTS: "It feels like my arm is popping out of joint." "I feel a click."

EXAM: Extend your arm in the air like the Statue of Liberty; now bring the arm back as if you're going to throw a football. Is there pain and resistance? Is there a sense of apprehension?

THERAPY: See Med Unit, page 166.

2. Rotator Cuff Syndrome/Bursitis

COMMENTS: "Doc, it hurts me when I put my jacket on. It's painful to reach behind me, or overhead."

EXAM: Put your arm straight out to your side with your thumb down and hold it there. Contrast the sensation you experience in the shoulder with that of your other shoulder in the same position. Is it painful? Reach around behind your body to remove your wallet. If you're a woman reach around to unhook your bra. Does that provide a serious twinge on the afflicted side? Take a can of soup and place it on the highest shelf in the kitchen. Does that hurt to do? Is the pain dull and throbbing, like a toothache in the shoulder?

THERAPY: See Med Unit, page 166.

3. AC Joint Problems

COMMENTS: "I feel a grinding."

EXAM: Press downward with your fingers on the raised bony bump on your shoulder, found roughly in the middle. Is there pain? Attempt to pull your arm crosswise across your chest. Is there pain?

THERAPY: See Med Unit, page 166.

4. *Biceps Tendonitis*

COMMENTS: "I have trouble carrying bags."

EXAM: holding a household weight of about five pounds in one hand (a full bag of ice or a bag of flour, for example, will work fine), attempt to curl the weight toward your body, as if your were doing biceps curls. Is there pain? Is it a dull pain?

THERAPY: See Med Unit, page 167.

5. *Muscular Aches and Pains of the Shoulder*

(These do not technically relate to the shoulder joint, but are often mistaken for shoulder problems.)

COMMENTS: "I feel a deep stiffness." "There's a pain in my shoulder muscle that goes halfway up the back of my neck." "I feel a deep, searing pain in my upper back." "If I rub the sore spot, it tends to feel better."

THERAPY: See Med Unit, page 167.

And now, as we say good-bye to the engineering marvel of the shoulder, I'd like to close the chapter with mention of a specific malady that is so compelling, dramatic, and close to my heart that it has its own specific name: Gorelick's Syndrome.

Gorelick's Syndrome

My childhood friend Abe Gorelick and his brothers all suffer from Gorelick's Syndrome, a very specific, sad, and life-changing malady, limited mainly to high school, but with implications in the wider world. The syndrome struck down every one of the Gorelick boys in turn, and in the very same way. Each of them—Bob, Walt, and Abe—were the best athletes in their class until the syndrome hit, and afterward took up math, law, and physics, in that order.

Gorelick's Syndrome struck Abe one afternoon in high school, where he was the local phenom pitcher. As adults we tend to forget just how intensely fought and coveted were those moments in bantam pinstripes, when we hurled and batted and slid into home, covered all over in clouds of glory in our own minds (or, if we were women, scored field hockey goals or threw the baton). Abe was a hot athlete—one of the most naturally talented young hurlers in the history of the school. Then one day, everything changed. Abe was starting against the "Mountain Lions," the dreaded division champs from one town over. At the beginning of the game, Abe was his usual stellar self, fanning six batters in row, and scattering a handful of weak dribblers and pop flies. Unfortunately for Abe, he had thrown tons of balls during batting practice in the days before the game, and he was still a skinny fifteen-year-old, without the reserves of muscular toughness that come with the secondary spurt of growth. Abe began struggling late in the fourth inning, and by the sixth, it was obvious that he was beginning to lose his trademark laser control—the first sign of fatigue in a pitching arm. Indifferent to Abe's fatigue, the coach, Randy "Hang 'em High" Calhoun, was adamant—this was a division tournament, after all, and Abe had gutted out a hundred difficult games before, so there was no reason to think this day would be any different. The coach was wrong—dead wrong. Some awful biomechanical alchemy took place in Abe's shoulder out there that day, and the result, by the end of game, was a vicious case of "hangdog" as we called it—a total limpness of the pitching arm. Gorelick's syndrome had struck—with gale force. Though Abe continued to pitch for another year, he was never the same. His fastball now wobbled weakly on invisible breezes, and his pitches dipped when they should have risen, and hung beckoning in the strike zone, ready to be murdered. Having endured the indignity of being "sent down" to the junior varsity, he taught the coach a lesson by walking a record seventeen batters in a row against an archrival team. Booed off the diamond, he grew a mustache, and in the way of high schoolers, spent a lot of time pretending to be someone else.

I've since examined Abe's shoulder—yes, we're still friends—and determined that what he did was to simply throw the shoulder out of joint. In medical parlance, he became a subluxer. Instead of the joint stably being there, it popped out repeatedly when torqued. A doctor could have tightened that up in a jiffy—with therapy, anti-inflammatories, and if necessary, surgery. But the key is that Abe *didn't* go to a doctor. He was afraid, most likely. And as a result, grew up with a strength-impaired right arm.

Gorelick's syndrome goes by many names. As do injuries to the shoulder. The key is seeking treatment aggressively and intelligently. But if you're still with me, I have to assume you're not only aggressive but intelligent too.

3

Hip, Thigh, and Groin

In 1992, I ran the New York Marathon. It was my third of these grueling events, and I was already familiar with its particular difficulties and joys. For those who don't know, the running of a marathon is not a snap decision. No one simply ups and runs twenty-six-plus miles on a lark, unless they're being chased by African killer bees. A marathon is normally preceded by a long training period. How long? If you want to run the marathon correctly, without injuring yourself, you have to live a lifestyle around the marathon for anywhere from four to eight months preceding the event. During this period, your diet changes: you eat more and more often, and increase the amount of complex carbohydrates in your meals. Your workouts and stretching become sports-specific: legs, hips, and feet. You grow very cognizant of hydration on a daily basis. Six hours before your daily run you begin thinking. How am I going to beat the elements? Have I drunk enough water? What equipment am I going to use to be sure I'm not injured? And so, day by day, the training for the marathon itself becomes a way of life.

In my case, I found myself regularly increasing my daily mileage during runs and worked with a stretching coach whose hands-on intervention increased my range of motion by about 15–20 percent. As the race day drew near I felt what I always felt: a mix of caution and excitement. Excitement that I'd be getting my report card at last, after excessive training. And caution, because one never knows if one's body is ready or not, despite all the training.

I had, as I said, run two marathons already, but each of those was like going to school—in each of them I found a whole new range of things to know in terms of pacing, controlling anxiety, timing, hydrating, and—why not say it—even going to the bathroom. The point being, I was no more certain of the outcome on my third marathon than I'd been of my first.

Race day happened at last. The weather was hot and sunny—which was both good and bad. Good because often your muscles work well in warmer weather, bad for the obvious reason that you sweat heavily. The race began: I felt light on my feet and was moving well. Eighteen miles in, I knew I was running a good race, knew I would not hit the wall, because I'd done my homework, and was prepared. The wall is a kind of metabolic crash, which you experience either from improper training or from running a race in such a way that you prematurely deplete your glycogen or muscle fuel. At such moments the pain and discomfort rise to levels that are beyond description. You want only that someone make it stop—even with a bullet in the brain if necessary. I had hit the wall before, and knew what it was about. But I felt no walls in my future just then. That's because I was in the *zone*.

Books have been written about it; athletes talk about it constantly. There are even TV commercials that use it as a selling point. What is the zone? In each sport it's different, but generally speaking, the zone is the apex of body awareness, a feeling of being "at oneness" with your physical self that requires nearly religious or spiritual terminology to describe. In my case, that day of the marathon, the zone was an uncanny sense of participation in my own body: a heightened consciousness of the blood pumping

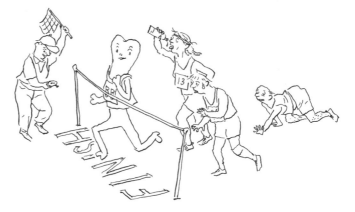

"The great thing about being a cartoon is I don't have to worry about dehydration and leg cramps."

through my arteries, my muscles sliding in their sheaths, my bones flexing with every step I took. The feeling was one of joy in living that is one of the very reasons that marathoners run marathons. Every sport has its peak moments—the perfect drive in golf; the three-point jump-shot swish in basketball; the cannon crosscourt in tennis—but the marathon differs from these in that its peak moment lasts for minutes at a time. For minutes and maybe even hours, that is, the body seems to slip its mortal limits and become pure energy, joy in motion. I was probably actually smiling when I stepped in a pothole and felt a searing knifelike stab on the back of the hamstring, which quickly rocketed up my leg to the insertion at the pelvis. I clutched my leg, gritted my teeth, and finished the race—but badly—limping across the finish line wearing my martian-invader face, and out of commission for eight weeks afterward. The peculiar pain of a strained hamstring resembles that of having your butt torched with a Zippo. No fun at all. So much for the zone.

ANATOMY

The hip joint is a ball and socket joint, like the shoulder, but in the stripped-down economy version, without the engineering genius of the shoulder, and therefore without the range of motion. Terminating at the hip is a braid of some of the largest muscles in the body: those of the thigh, which lead from the hip to the knee. These muscular structures enwrap the thighbone front and back and circumferentially, and give the body its propulsive power. The quadriceps muscle on the front are composed of four different muscles—the rectus femoris, the vastus lateralis, the vastus intermedius, and the vastus medialis (Fig. 3.1). Of these, the rectus femoris is the only one that crosses two joints, the hip and knee, and as such, is the most commonly injured. The muscles behind, known as the hamstrings, are actually three different muscle groups—the semitendonosus, biceps femoris, and semimembranosus. The muscles on the inner and outer parts of the thigh are called the adductors and abductors, respectively (Fig. 3.2).

The hip joint can be thought of as the sentinel or guard of the lower half of the body. It's not flashy; it's not glamorous. It's a workhorse, a Clydesdale in fact—massive, simple, and obedient. Large in scale, it doesn't get

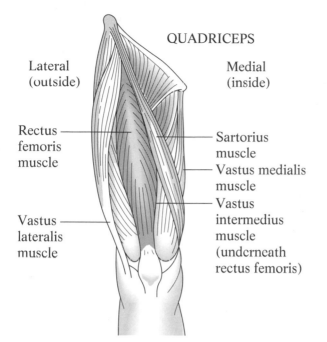

QUADRICEPS

Lateral
(outside)

Medial
(inside)

Rectus
femoris
muscle

Sartorius
muscle

Vastus medialis
muscle

Vastus
intermedius
muscle
(underneath
rectus femoris)

Vastus
lateralis
muscle

Fig. 3.1 Front view of thigh muscle.

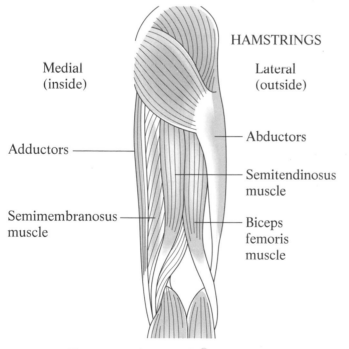

HAMSTRINGS

Medial
(inside)

Lateral
(outside)

Abductors

Adductors

Semitendinosus
muscle

Semimembranosus
muscle

Biceps
femoris
muscle

Fig. 3.2 Back view of thigh muscle.

injured often. Rarely does it complain, except from stiffness. The hip is a very stabilized strong joint, which requires a huge amount of trauma to pull from its socket. Take my marathon mishap, for example: I had injured not the joint itself, that day, but had damaged the hamstring at the place where it attached to the pelvis near the hip. To actually damage the powerful ball and socket of the hip requires something like a motorcycle accident—which is why, as in my case, the accidents are mainly muscular rather than *osseus*, or bony. But when the hip goes, it goes big.

INJURIES

From a diagnostic point of view, hip difficulties are peculiarly challenging because the hip is in the middle of so many organ systems—abdominal and gynecological. My Colombo-like faculties are often taxed to their maximum as I work to zero in on the problems. Hernias and the quadriceps attachment, for example, are very very close, and are often misdiagnosed. When I say "attachment," I mean the place where the muscle strands attach to the bone. As befits this crucial area, the muscle has swelled into a tough and fibrous bundle at this point, the better to make the connection. Obviously, any trauma to the muscle at large, will travel up to the point where the muscle—moving—attaches to the static place: the pelvis, in this case.

Here are some typical groups of muscles that terminate at the hip and that get strained during athletics: The **quadriceps** muscles, which are the big muscles in the front of the thigh; the butt muscles or **gluteus maximus**; the **hamstring** muscles, which are in the back of the thigh; the **abductor** and **abductor** muscles, which allow your leg to move to the side. All of these injure themselves in a similar way.

For people who don't warm up and plunge right into aggressive sports activities like sprinting, tennis, or touch football, beware! This is one of the areas of the body most sensitive to abrupt workouts without warm-up. The result of not allowing muscles the proper warm-up can be chronic tendonitis problems—microtears of the tendons that terminate or originate at the pelvis, which produce a long-term, gradual, insidious pain that can be as damaging, finally, as an outright rip. Typical hip tendonitis problems involve the hip flexor muscle on the front of the thigh and the adductor muscle. All long-term pain in the hip joint should be looked into, and x-rayed, to rule out degenerative arthritis, stress fracture, or possibly a congenital dislocation.

OTHER HIP (AND UPPER LEG) AILMENTS

Bruises

Obviously, with a big muscle like the thigh exposed to the bangs and cleats and elbows of the world, you're going to suffer some serious bruising to the tissues now and again if you play sports regularly. Everyone knows bruises (or contusions as they're called in med-speak) and knows when what they have is serious, or a garden-variety black-and-blue. One of the dangers of a hip bruise is that if it is deep enough, and accompanied by enough intramuscular bleeding, it can cause calcium deposits to form, a condition called *myositis ossificans*, which can impede muscle function, and is very difficult to treat. The other thing to bear in mind with hip and thigh bruises is that, due to gravity, the subcutaneous or below-the-skin bleeding can travel a bit. You can bang your hip and find those lovely sunset bruise colors ending up on your thigh. The culprit in such cases is gravity, nothing more.

Hip Pointer

This is second cousin to hip contusion and takes place when the *iliac crest*, the bony part of the pelvis whose rim can be felt on either side of the waistline, gets bruised. Hip pointers are commonly caused by the kinds of direct impact seen in a football tackle and hockey slam, and can be difficult to treat, because the large muscles that terminate there put the area under constant stress. If treated correctly, with ice and compression, the more serious side effects can usually be avoided, and the injury will resolve itself within two to three weeks.

Bo Jackson's Ball and Socket

Remember Bo Jackson? Well, Bo might have known baseball, and football too, but he didn't know what would happen when he was body-slammed into the AstroTurf one fine afternoon. The impact of that violent tackle was centered entirely on the hip, which, as a result of the force of the blow, became necrotic. In layman's terms, blood stopped flowing to his hip, and the bone began to die. It needed to be replaced. This is a very rare accident, and will most likely not trouble the weekend athletes and joggers.

More common than violent trauma to the hip are overuse problems. **Bursitis of the hip** is a frequent one. The problem in hip bursitis centers not in the hip itself, but in the bursa, the little tough lubricating disc where the muscles attach, which becomes inflamed. Bursitis of the hip is often caused by sudden weight gain, and is therefore a problem during pregnancy.

Old age also brings it particular difficulties to the hips. The wear and tear of a lifetime often centers in the hip joints, which become so worn away that they need to be replaced. Unfortunately, people tend to think of getting their joints replaced these days as something akin to buying a new car: should I get it in pink or purple, with a sunroof or with air-conditioning? An accompanying delusion is that a person with a hip replacement can be every bit the athlete he or she was before. Not true. Hip replacements are a last resort, and will allow you to have a life, but not a fully restored athletic life.

Groin Pull

The groin pull, as it's commonly known, is a strain or rupture of the adductor longus muscle, which runs from the pubic bone to the inner part of the thigh, and allows you to swing your leg inward. These muscles are particularly developed in professional jockeys, who spend their time on horseback pressing their legs inward for dear life! A groin pull is easily diagnosed by attempting to pull the leg inward. Pain and difficulty while doing so are surefire signs of a pull. Treatment for groin pulls is almost always nonsurgical, and involves rest, anti-inflammatories, and, if the muscle is torn, a physical therapy program to ensure minimum buildup of scar tissue during the healing phase.

Muscle Imbalance

Another physical difficulty that often makes itself felt at the hip is *muscle imbalance.* Over a lifetime many people develop bad habits of favoring one side or aspect of their bodies, often unconsciously. This can have psychological reasons (as in wanting to protect a body part; I have often noticed that women who want to protect their breasts, stoop over, for example), or it can be congenital in origin. In either case, the strains and torques of this kind of compensation often end up knocking at the door of the hip, with painful results.

What is all this leading to? A simple statement: For all athletics involving the hip, stretching is probably more important than for any other area of the body. Stretching the hip is not easy, because it is such a large, powerful joint, so entrenched among its muscles and difficult to access. Men, in particular, tend to be tight in this area. My friends who teach yoga tell me that when they do hip stretches in class the men often complain that they have "a lot of rage" in their hips. I'm not sure what this means exactly, but I find it an interesting concept. In any case, the message is clear: If you do anything involving running or jumping, be sure to stretch long and hard before starting out. Consult Appendix B for details about stretching.

Now that you have an understanding of the anatomy of the hip, thigh, and groin and their most common injuries, let's continue on to Part One of the Bio-Point Exam.

The BIO-POINT Exam

Hip, Thigh, and Groin

PART ONE

Question 1

Is there any deformity in the afflicted area? Look in the mirror and if possible compare the affected and the unaffected side. Is there a lack of symmetry?
If "yes," see a doctor immediately.
If "no," read on.

Question 2

Is there a severe limitation in your range of motion? Are you incapable of performing basic household tasks with the afflicted extremity?
If "yes," see a doctor immediately.
If "no," read on.

Question 3

Is there any sign of extensive or excessive swelling?
If "yes," see a doctor immediately.
If "no," read on.

Question 4

Are you afflicted with severe weakness in the injured body part? Do you have difficulty, for example, climbing stairs?
If "yes," see a doctor immediately.
If "no," read on.

Question 5

Was a loud "pop" heard at the time of the injury?
If "yes," see a doctor immediately.
If "no," read on.

Whew! You're still with me! That's very good news because it means your injury may fall within the guidelines of what is treatable at home. What I'm going to do now is to zero in on your problem and attempt to make a more accurate diagnosis. Look at the accompanying illustration and touch the area where your pain or discomfort is most specific and localized. Note the number and the name of the injury (on the illustration) that corresponds with this area. Based on the area of pain you've indicated, this is likely to be the correct diagnosis. However, remember that injuries often overlap! Therefore, I recommend that you don't leap to any

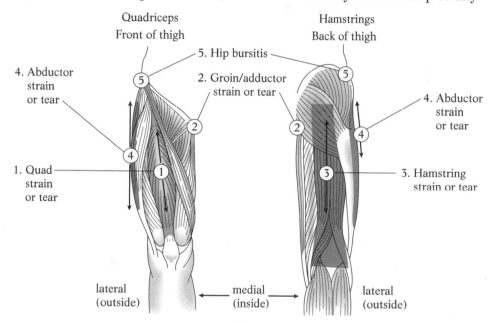

conclusion. Follow through by doing *all* of the Bio-Point Exams. This will ensure the most accurate and informed assessment of your injury. To help guide you in determining your own injury, each exam includes typical comments from patients suffering from that particular injury. After each exam, the page number of the corresponding Med Unit is given. The Med Units are in Appendix A. By following the Med Unit instructions, you can begin treating your injury immediately, keeping close track of your progress as you go.

1. Quad Strain or Tear

COMMENTS: "I heard a pop and felt my leg give out." "I have pain when I walk and run."

EXAM: Sit in a chair. Bring your knee to your chest while resisting the upward pull of your leg with the downward push of your knee. Do you feel pain in the center of the quadriceps? Is it a toothachelike pain? Is it a sharp pain?

THERAPY: See Med Unit, pages 167–168.

2. Groin/Adductor Strain or Tear

COMMENTS: Same as Quad Strain or Tear.

EXAM: Sit in a chair. Bring your knee to your chest, then attempt to squeeze you thigh inward while pushing outward with your hand. Is there a toothachelike pain in your inner thigh? Is it a sharp pain?

THERAPY: see Med unit, pages 167–168.

3. Hamstring Strain or Tear

COMMENTS: Same as Quad Strain or Tear.

EXAM: Lie on your stomach. Bring your heel into your buttock (as if you were performing a hamstring curl) while a partner applies resistance with his or her hand. Is there pain in the buttock or down the back of the thigh?

THERAPY: See Med Unit, pages 167–168.

4. Abductor Strain or Tear

COMMENTS: Same as Quad Strain or Tear.

EXAM: Sit in a chair. Bring your knee into your chest, then attempt to push your thigh outward while pushing inward with your hand. Is there a toothachelike pain in your outer thigh? Is it a sharp pain?

THERAPY: See Med Unit, pages 167–168.

5. Hip Bursitis

COMMENTS: "I have pain and swelling in my outer hip." "I feel a snapping in my hip." "I feel pain radiating down my thigh."

EXAM: Do you feel pain especially in area 5 on the illustration?

THERAPY: See Med Unit, page 168.

6. Snapping Hip

This is a condition in which one of one of the tendons, on either the outside or the inside of the hip, snaps over the bone.

THERAPY: If this describes your condition, you should see a doctor.

4

Elbow

Every once in a while we read about an athlete who is able to upset the actuarial applecart by playing with excellence well past his prime. Among baseball pitchers, there are several recent examples who come to mind, among them Nolan Ryan and Tommy John. Often the reason they last as long as they do is because of the perfection of their form. In the case of Tommy John, who retired a few years ago in his early forties, he not only possessed superb form, but also got an assist from modern medicine—specifically, surgery on an ulnar collateral ligament tear, which is as common as rain among baseball players. Up until the time of John's surgery, it was also a surefire career-ender. He was the first pitcher in major league baseball to benefit from modern surgical techniques, which allowed the injury—to the main stabilizing ligament of the elbow—to be properly diagnosed, treated, and eliminated. After the surgery, when reporters would ask him, "Mr. John, you're thirty-eight years old, how many years do you think you have left?" John would brandish the reconstructed elbow, and say cheerfully, "yeah, but my arm is only *three years* old!"

The elbow belongs to that category of easily ignored things like indoor plumbing and elasticized waistbands, without which life would be unthinkable. Part of the reason people pay little attention to the elbow is because the elbow, on the surface, is an unsexy customer. A hinge joint whose role in life is the boring one of opening and shutting like a Swiss Army knife, the elbow hasn't the complex hydraulic genius of the knee, nor the free-range suavness of the shoulder. Most people know it as the pointy spots in the middle of their arms. And yet, biomechanically, the elbow is as beautiful as a swan. To continue the metaphor, the elbow is in a certain sense like a swan swimming. Outwardly, everything is calm, but just below the surface, things are boiling—cartilaginous plates are crunching, and tendons and ligaments are sliding through bone tunnels like something out of the film *Anaconda*. This is because of the elbow's specialized—let's hear it all together—anatomy.

ANATOMY

Muscularly speaking, the elbow is the Grand Central Station of joints. Eight muscles terminate there, a veritable downtown of quick-twitch fibers. The biceps, the triceps, and a variety of forearm flexor muscles all call the elbow home. Three major arm bones also end up there: the humerus, ulna and radius (see Fig 4.1). The biceps attach to the radius bone in the forearm and permit the arm to bend and flex. The triceps attach to the ulna in the forearm and permit extension and straightening of the arm—in addition to allowing the wrist to turn clockwise (see Fig. 4.2). Ligaments, the body's rubber girders, hold the whole structure together and allow it to perform its function.

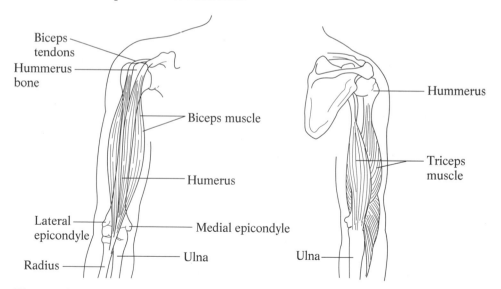

Fig. 4.1 Front view of arm and elbow.   **Fig. 4.2 Back view of arm and elbow.**

The entire wrist and finger flexion and extension begin at the elbow—meaning that the tiniest flick of your finger travels all the way up to the elbow. And the elbow, on a larger scale, is the place where the fulcral stresses generated by the arms are centered. Imagine a pitcher pitching. The arm is flung high over the head, and then jerked downward from the shoulder. But what gives that fastball it's real whip-cracking speed is the secondary flexing of the elbow, which both stops the initial downward motion and accelerates it at the same time: strike! The shock of stopping the movement is the elbow's responsibility. In swimming, pitching, tennis, golf, and fly casting, the initial movement is initiated by the shoulder, and then both braked and accelerated by the elbow.

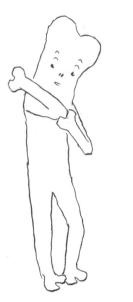

"The doctor says it's a biomechanical marvel, but it looks like a plain old elbow to to me."

The elbow, fortunately, is not a joint that wears out often, and is far less likely to suffer from arthritis than, for example, the knees or the hip. Its problems have more to do with overuse injuries to the tendons and ligaments that connect in the elbow, rather than the biology of the bone itself. Nonethless, the elbow has a separate chapter to itself in this book, not because so many different things go wrong with it, but because when things do go wrong with it, they are so often the same: tendonitis, in a word. Or in two words, *tennis elbow*.

INJURIES

Tennis Elbow

This is the big one, ladies and gentlemen, the mother of all overuse injuries, the Eiffel Tower of inflammations. Lateral humeral epicondylitis is

Parent's Advisory

"Little League elbow" is a tendonitis-related inflammatory twinge of the elbow, which occurs in pint-size hurlers and hitters. Caused by the powerful downward snap of the ball-release, it goes to the weakest point in the child's arm—the growth cartilage—where it can cause permanent damage. If caught early enough, the damaged cartilage can reattach. Remember: if your children are complaining of elbow pain from throwing, it's a potentially serious condition. See a doctor immediately. And in the meantime, have them give up pitching and head for the outfield fast.

the way they say it in Latin. "My elbow is killing me, Doc" is the way my patients say it. And they say it an awful lot. They come streaming into my office from the tennis, squash, and racquetball courts, touching their elbows, holding their damaged wings to their chests. The boom in recreational sports has sponsored a related boom in elbow overuse injuries, but tennis elbow, in fact, is a catchall term for *elbow tendonitis*, whose causes run the gamut from housepainting to baby-carrying, to even, in certain cases, using the computer.

The first thing I tell my wincing patients is that though tennis elbow injuries may be painful, they're rarely dangerous if caught early and treated properly. The second thing I do is ask them some detailed questions about the repetitive motions they make in a day. As with all joint injuries, interactivity plays a key role, and whether it's lifting weights, the garage door, or moving hundreds of pounds of water as you swim in the pool, the complex web of motions that forms a day's activity must be examined to see if they contribute to the injury-syndrome. Often, in overuse injuries, there is an obsessive component to the problem—a repetitive motion that has simply tuckered out the joint.

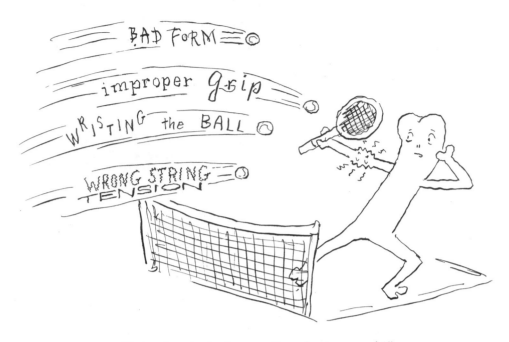

"I simply asked why my elbow hurt so much!"

The good news about "pure" tennis elbow is that it's easily improved by changes in racket, grip, string tension, and or the swing itself. The main cause of tennis elbow is the players—through fatigue or bad instruction—"arming" or "wristing" the ball—trying to muscle it across the net with their forearms, rather than through the torque of their shoulders. This undue stress on arm muscles not intended for this purpose transmits the shock right back up the bones and muscles to the nearest hinge joint, which happens to be our favorite orthopedic piece of Swiss cutlery, the—you guessed it—elbow. If any of these conditions develop, reexaming your technique—and possibly a lesson with the local pro—is as important as any of the other medical treatments.

A related version of tennis elbow is golf elbow, which irritates the tendons of the inner side of the elbow. The same inflammation patterns occur, but golf elbow sometimes has even worse inflammation because you are not hitting a soft ball with pliant strings, as in tennis, but whacking a hard little pellet with a steel rod (or sometimes, let's face it, whacking the ground itself). The impact, accordingly, is more traumatic.

Form

I've already given you a brief lecture on form, and have explained how correcting your form by a millimeter can spawn enormous positive consequences in your overall athletic functioning. Need more examples? Take Bjorn Borg, one of the first of the tennis power players, who combined sprinter's speed with diabolically strong ground strokes. Why did he retire at an early age? As a casualty of poor form, his body was already wearing out. Take a friend of mine, a dancer at one of the country's leading ballet companies. Why, at the age of twenty-nine, did the joints of his body begin suddenly clacking like the castanets in a flamenco music? You guessed it, poor form. Both of these two were natural athletes, but both practiced their athletic art without worrying about the toll it was taking on their underlying physical structure. Their form was off, and as a result, each drew heavily from their body's natural well of performance. Up until around age thirty, you can cheat by relying on the body's self-replenishing natural processes. But if you haven't replenished the well of the body by that age, and have been drawing heavily on it, it will—as it did in these two examples—run dry, and you'll have to hang up your tap shoes.

OTHER ELBOW INJURIES

Snapping of the Ulnar Nerve

It's not a very common problem but it's common enough to be included here. The ulnar bone is the technical term for what most people call the "funny bone." It contains a strip of exposed nerve, which fits in a groove in the bottom of the elbow and is very vulnerable to being hit or stressed or overused. Multiple traumatic events or congenital abnormality can lead to a chronic condition. The symptoms are distinct from tennis elbow, and they are unpleasant: a lack of sensation, potential muscular weakness, and pain and shooting electrical hotshots going down to the pinkie and the fourth finger.

Bone Chips

No, these are not a barbecue additive to flavor meat. They are what happens when you either grind your elbow or shatter it. In either case, tiny chips (called by surgeons "joint mice" for their tendency to scurry around the elbow, moving from place to place) are the result. Obviously, they impede motion. You often hear of them being removed from the arms of major league pitchers. To illustrate the problem for my patients—who, as usual, of course, want nothing more than to throw away their slings and casts and sprint back to the tennis court and golf course—I go to the door of my examining room, stick a pen in the hinge of it, and then try to close it. Aside from costing me a fortune in Bics, this shows very simply why they can't extend their arms: the wedge of a bone chip is in the way of the joint. In such cases as this, there is no choice but to go in surgically—to that very small space within the elbow—and remove the chips.

GENERAL TREATMENT FOR ELBOW PAIN AND TENDONITIS

In general, all inflammatory injuries falling under this category are treated the same way. There are joint-specific treatments, however. An injection of cortisone, for example, is particularly useful for elbows. If it's a question of tennis elbow, then a consultation with the clubhouse pro about your form is in order. Otherwise, rest, ice, cessation or change in activity are indicated.

When it comes to surgery, the elbow, like other joints, has benefited from the arthroscopic revolution. Joint longevity has been increased and healing intervals have been shortened. All healing comes from energizing, nutrient-rich blood flow. A new technique, which often gives great results, is to lightly drill into the mating surface of the bones, allowing blood flow and the potential for a new smooth surface to form, thereby extending the life of the joint.

Now that you have an understanding of the anatomy of the elbow and its most common injuries, let's continue on to Part One of the Bio-Point Exam.

The BIO-POINT Exam

E l b o w

PART ONE

Question 1

Is there any deformity in the afflicted area? Look in the mirror and if possible compare the affected and the unaffected side. Is there a lack of symmetry?
If "yes," see a doctor immediately.
If "no," read on.

Question 2

Is there a severe limitation in your range of motion? Are you incapable of performing basic household tasks with the afflicted extremity?
If "yes," see a doctor immediately.
If "no," read on.

Question 3

Is there any sign of extensive or excessive swelling?
If "yes," see a doctor immediately.
If "no," read on.

Question 4

Are you afflicted with severe weakness in the injured body part? Do you have difficulty, for example, gripping a can?
If "yes," see a doctor immediately.
If "no," read on.

Question 5

Was a loud "pop" heard at the time of the injury?
If "yes," see a doctor immediately.
If "no," read on.

PART TWO

Whew! You're still with me! That's very good news because it means your injury may fall within the guidelines of what is treatable at home. What

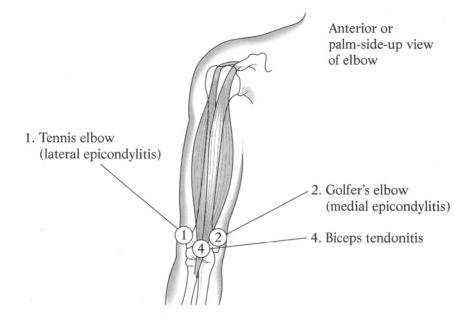

Anterior or palm-side-up view of elbow

1. Tennis elbow (lateral epicondylitis)

2. Golfer's elbow (medial epicondylitis)

4. Biceps tendonitis

I'm going to do now is to zero in on your problem and attempt to make a more accurate diagnosis. Look at the accompanying illustration and touch the area where your pain or discomfort is most specific and localized. Note the number and the name of the injury (on the illustration) that corresponds with this area. Based on the area of pain you've indicated, this is likely to be the correct diagnosis. However, remember that injuries often overlap! Therefore, I recommend that you don't leap to any conclusions. Follow through by doing *all* of the Bio-Point Exams. This will ensure the most accurate and informed assessment of your injury. To help guide you in determining your own injury, each exam includes typical com-

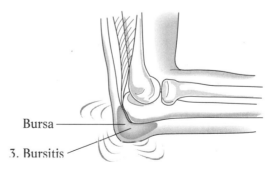

Bursa

3. Bursitis

Side view of elbow

ments from patients suffering from that particular injury. After each exam, the page number at the corresponding Med Unit is given. The Med Units are in Appendix A. Note: If no Med Unit is given, immediate medical attention is advised—since this condition cannot be treated at home. By following the Med Unit instructions, you can begin treating your injury immediately, keeping close track of your progress as you go.

1. Tennis Elbow (Lateral Epicondylitis)

COMMENTS: "I have difficulty picking up objects, especially with my arm straight."

EXAM: Extend your arm straight out in front of you with your palm facing up as if you're signaling STOP! Then attempt to push the palm downward against resistance (you can either use your other hand or push against a wall). Is there pain in the outer elbow?

THERAPY: See Med Unit, page 168.

2. Golfer's Elbow (Medical Epicondylitis)

COMMENTS: Same as Tennis Elbow.

EXAM: Do the exact opposite as for the Tennis Elbow exam. Extend your arm straight out in front of you (palm facing down). Curl your wrist downward (fingers toward the floor). Attempt to bring your hand back up against resistance (again, you can use your other hand). Is there pain in the inner elbow? Does the pain radiate?

OTHER COMMENTS: This evil twin brother of tennis elbow can strike as a result of a variety of sporting activities, aside from golf, including baseball and track and field events. If left untreated, the nearby ulnar nerve may be damaged. Pain and numbness typically radiate through to the pinkie finger.

THERAPY: See Med Unit, page 169.

3. Bursitis

COMMENTS: "There's a lump on the back of my elbow." "Is this cancer?"

"How did this get here?"

EXAM: Squeeze the mass at the end of your elbow. Does it feel like a water balloon?

OTHER COMMENTS: Elbow bursitis may or may not be the result of trauma. If a trauma has occurred, see a doctor to rule out fracture.

THERAPY: If no trauma has occurred, see Med Unit, page 169.

4. Biceps Tendonitis

COMMENTS: "My elbow hurts when I try to lift things." "My elbow hurts when I lift weights."

EXAM: Press on the biceps tendon in the middle of the elbow (see illustration on page 59). Is there pain? Attempt to curl the elbow toward you (as if you were performing a biceps curl or lifting a bucket). Is there pain?

THERAPY: See Med Unit, page 169.

5. Elbow Sprain

COMMENTS: "I have pain all over my elbow with pronounced stiffness." "I feel a tingling, numb sensation."

THERAPY: See a doctor. There is the possibility of a fracture or nerve damage.

6. Bone Chip (Osteochondritis Dissecans) or Bone Spur

COMMENTS: "I feel a locking or popping in my elbow." "I can't fully extend my elbow without pain."

EXAM: Flex your elbow slowly. Is there an audible or palpable pop? Is there a feeling of your elbow "catching"?

OTHER COMMENTS: The bone chip is the bane of pitchers.

THERAPY: See a doctor if these describe your symptoms. Surgery may be necessary.

5

Hand and Wrist

Hands are intriguing indexes of the personality and life of their owner, reflecting both the genetic endowment of that person and the way they've lived their life. Are their hands beat-up and scarred from manual labor? Are the nails bitten from nervousness? Stained with tobacco? Are the hands pampered and soft from a life indoors? Everyone knows a butcher with thick and meaty hands, the pianist with long, thin fingers. Anthropologist friends often tell me that in their travels around the world, the first thing they look at when they meet indigenous people is their hands (and feet), as a way of getting a quick "read" on these persons' essential physical makeup.

I'm no anthropologist, but I share their fascination with the function of the hands. The five fingers of the human hand are gifted with an extremely high ratio of nerve endings to muscle fibers, and are animated by tiny muscles of orchestral complexity. The reason for this is that the hand is called upon to per-

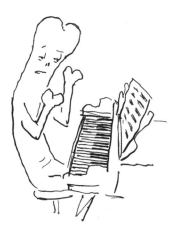

"God, cartoonists are so lazy!"

form a wider variety of tasks than any other part of the body. From the pinpoint control of a blazing fastball to the sheer power to crank a stuck lid off a jar; from the delicacy to thread a needle to the levering of a body up a sheer rock face, the hands are that part of us most involved with negotiating between ourselves and our external environment.

The wrist brokers the connection of the delicate phalanges (fingers) of the hand to the powerful muscles of the upper arm, and allows all the power of the biceps and tendons to be routed through a swiveling arc of about 160 degrees. The wrist, unfortunately, is rather a brittle joint, and often bears the brunt for overuse injuries—in addition, of course, to the trauma of falls and sprains.

Those of you with babies or young children are probably familiar with something called the "parachute response." This is the instinctual reaction of even tiny babies to a perceived fall. They splay their arms and wrists to cushion the impact and protect the face. The response continues in various forms into adulthood, and is one reason, among many, why people falling off of horses, or tripping while jogging or sprinting, or getting thrown to the ground in a football tackle so often end up with broken wrists: the hands come out to ward off the impact, and before they know what they're doing, they've got a broken bone.

ANATOMY

Remember the movie *The Terminator*, where Arnold's synthetic skin is peeled back to reveal the glittering metallic joints of his hand? The terminator's anatomy was accurate as far as it went, but it was a kiddie version of the real thing. The musculoskeletal architecture that allows us, Homo sapiens, to be able to grasp, is among the body's most obvious works of genius.

But that genius is not simple; it's complex. The hand is rooted in the wrist joint, a hinge joint that connects the forearm and the wrist bones. This joint is found between the end of the ulna and radius bones of the arm, and the carpal bones of the wrist ("carpal" as in "tunnel syndrome": on the palm side of the wrist is the troublesome carpal tunnel, home to the median nerve). To these carpal bones are attached another series of bones called the metacarpals, which form the palm of the hand. On top of them are the phalanges as they're known, the long jointed tapering bones that comprise our actual fingers. The thumb, miracle of free-range motion, has its own saddle-shaped joint (see Figs 5.1 and 5.2).

The wrist is operated through the muscles of the forearm. Hands and fingers have twenty-seven muscles, each of them calibrated to fantastically fine microtolerances, and the thumb has eight separate muscles and tendons of its own. The next time you give a "thumbs up," remember you're doing more than making an approving gesture. You're using the thenar and adductor muscles, plus the long flexor, abductor, and two extensor pollicis muscles!

The hand is covered with skin custom-fitted so that its density and elasticity changes from one part to another: loose on the back of the hand, tight on the palm. In addition, muscle creases along the palm allow for wide-ranging flexion of the fingers. A grid of nerves fans outward from the wrist, reaching its maximum density and sensitivity in the thumb and the first three fingers. The hands are powered through forearm muscle-tendons, which wind over and under the wrist and then split up to attach to the fingers. This is way, way beyond anything out of Hollywood special effects!

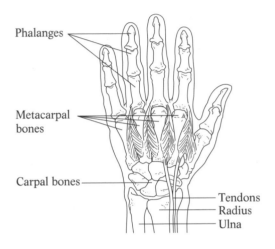

Fig. 5.1 Top (dorsal) view of hand and wrist.

Phalanges

Metacarpal bones

Carpal bones

Tendons
Radius
Ulna

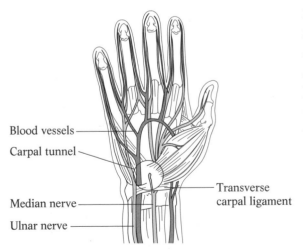

Fig. 5.2 Palm view of hand and wrist.

Blood vessels

Carpal tunnel

Median nerve

Ulnar nerve

Transverse carpal ligament

INJURIES

When it comes to sports, the hands(and wrists) come in for quite a beating. They are by far the limb of the body most injured in competitive sports. Strained and smashed, contused, jammed and broken, they bear the fate of those other extremities, the feet, but without the protective covering of a tough shoe. Hands also differ from the feet in that, when injured, they must be restored to perfect preinjury functioning. Even a slight malalignment will have deep, deep consequences for a limb as dependent on anatomical microtolerances as the hand. The foot, by comparison, is a more sturdy, plebian operation. If the five toes are Rockettes, the five fingers are prima ballerinas.

The wrist can be injured by the trauma of a fall, but is as often injured by repetitive-motion syndromes. These are commonly exacerbated by a weight involved in the motion: bowling with a heavy ball; throwing the javelin, practicing gymnastics, even, for that matter, using a jackhammer. All of these activities cause immense stress and potential overuse trauma to the wrist. The guy who goes out to his local driving range and whacks five buckets of golf balls without any previous practice and no sense of proper form, may congratulate himself for a good time, but he may also wake up in the middle of the night with a hand the size of an oven mitt: the wrist again, making its presence felt.

All of these overuse injuries, as common and troublesome as they are, pale in comparison to that other overuse injury, that quiet the injury that has caused umpteen millions of lost work days over the last few years, and spawned an industry of diagnosis and care all its own: *carpal tunnel syndrome.*

Carpal Tunnel Syndrome

No, this is not a shortcut to get to Hoboken, it is a pervasive inflammation, which is one of the most common species of what's called, in med-speak, "nerve entrapment." In such cases the central (or median) nerve riding up a tunnel through the middle of the wrist is "trapped" or compressed by swelling (Fig 5.3, p. 66). Pain and numbness soon follow. Carpal tunnel produces a characteristic discomfort on the radial side or thumb side of the hand.

The common wisdom about carpal tunnel is that it's limited to people who've spent too much time in front of the computer terminal, typing with their wrists unsupported. It's true that hardcore typists are far more prone to it than others, and that the computer, in addition to making Bill Gates as rich as God, has spawned a whole new class of sufferers. But carpal tunnel is not limited to computer users alone. Bike riders are often afflicted, and manufacturers have heeded their

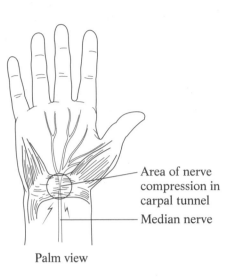

Area of nerve compression in carpal tunnel

Median nerve

Palm view

Fig. 5.3 Carpal tunnel syndrome with nerve being trapped in tunnel.

cries and redesigned handlebars to cut down on the incidence of it. Golfers get it. Meatcutters and textile workers get it. Musicians sometimes get it. Women can get it from the generalized swelling that accompanies pregnancy. People climbing their way to heaven on StairMasters get it. Anyone who grips something tightly for a long period of time risks getting it. It is not life-threatening, but it can create considerable discomfort if left untreated.

The typical treatment is (RICE) rest, ice, cessation of activity, and elevation and sometimes anti-inflammatories. Often, people simply need to stay away from the offending item: bike, computer, or stairMaster for a while. Special wrist splints are available,

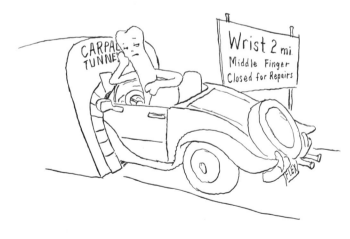

"They told me my swollen muscle car might get caught at Carpal Tunnel. Why didn't I buy Volkswagen?"

which immobilize the wrist in a helpful position. Sometimes a cortisone injection will do the trick. If not, surgery may be necessary to widen the blocked nerve canal. It should be remembered that not everyone who has numbness in his or her hand is suffering from carpal tunnel. There are potentially three or four sites of impingement of the nerve that animates the fingers and wrist. A test called an EMG or nerve conduction test can determine exactly where the problem is.

OTHER COMMON WRIST INJURIES

Tendonitis of the Wrist

The wrist is densely wound with tendons, any of which can potentially grow inflamed and cause difficulties. One of the more common types of wrist tendonitis has the name of a pricey French restaurant: *de Quervain's syndrome*. This is an inflammation that often occurs among players of racket sports, and is frequently seen among computer users to boot. A repetitive-motion injury, it is treated similarly to carpal tunnel syndrome, with rest, icing, cessation of activity, anti-inflammatories, or cortisone injection usually doing the trick.

You can get tendon twinges by the thumb, in the center of the wrist, on the outer part of the wrist, or by the base of the pinkie. Sports in which a repetitive snapping motion is important—baseball, golf, tennis, canoeing—generally leave the wrist open to trouble.

Diagnostically speaking, a doctor precedes by isolating the specific area of pain. This is called "point tender." If a person is "point tender" over the area where the tendon attaches to a specific bone of the wrist, then a specific treatment program for that inflamed tendon is put into motion. Again, surgery is rarely indicated for these kinds of tendonitis problems.

Jammed Finger

Have you ever noticed how often you see professional athletes playing with their fingers taped together during games? It never seems to damage their shooting percentages or pass reception either. Their fingers are taped either to ward off the worsening of a preexisting finger condition, or to stabilize an already damaged digit. Finger injuries are the bane of professional athletes, and the most common one of all—the one most likely to afflict the weekend athlete as well—is the "jammed finger."

In the nonathletic world, we call it a sprain, but among basketball, baseball, and football players, it's known as the jammed finger. Anatomically speaking, it is the result of a stretched and torn ligament. Medically speaking, it's unusually common. The jammed finger can occur in any sport, or even from a household fall or moment of physical awkwardness. It comes in three flavors: Grades I, II, and III, ranging from a 25 percent tear of the ligament to a full blown wall-to-wall rip. Due to the amount of nerves wound everywhich way through the fingers, it hurts like hell on wheels.

The severity of the ligament damage determines the healing pattern and recovery times. Sometimes ligament problems from jammed fingers can turn chronic, and require surgical reconstruction, which often leaves the fingers disfigured, but they mostly heal on their own. Though the ligaments of the finger joints are loose compared to others in the body (the better to allow all that wonderful hand-to-eye gripping and releasing), these ligaments are still strong enough to sometimes take a piece of bone with them when they tear. This is called an *avulsion fracture,* which requires conservative treatment including splinting or taping.

Dislocation

This is the next stage of severity for a jammed finger or a sprain. In this case, the bone is separated at the joint from another bone. Obviously, in such cases, soft tissue and ligamentous structures are severely damaged. Specifically damaged in such cases is a thing called the *volar plate,* which is a cartilage plate that spans the gap between bones. At moments of dislocation, he-man heroics that you commonly see when people pop the finger back in is precisely what you should **not** do, because if this is not done in exactly the right way, it can make matters much worse. As I've said, a dislocated finger is a finger that has suffered soft-tissue damage at the joint, and potentially fractured the bone. The treatment for this is to realign the finger and immobilize it until healed—better left to a professional.

Mallet Finger

This is a rip of the tendon at the tip of the finger, which causes the finger to flop into a characteristic mallet shape. It's also called "football jersey finger," because it is so often seen when tacklers grab onto a jersey to bring a runner down, and rip the top of the tendon of the finger in the process, sometimes breaking off a piece of the bone. It is also commonly caused by getting hit directly on the finger from a baseball or a volleyball. Unless there are broken bones involved, the treatment is immobilization in an extended position, to allow the ruptures to heal. This usually takes six to eight weeks. Most people do quite well with this treatment.

Ganglions/Cysts

Cysts occur all over the body, but they have a particular fondness for the wrist. Countless patients have come to me in fear over the sudden bulging protuberance on his or her wrist. Almost invariably, this is a benign cystic lesion, called a ganglion, and not the galloping cancer the patient fears. These can be treated with surgery if they become painful, or are cosmetically deforming. Fortunately, advances in medicine preclude what used to be done with wrist cysts in the 1700s: they were smashed with a heavy book, most often the Bible. You've heard of the phrase "Bible-thumping?" This certainly got rid of the cyst, but in the process, often broke many of the small bones of the joint.

Skiier's thumb

One of the most common of all ligament tears is the dreaded "skiiers thumb," a ripping of the ligament at the base of the thumb, where the thumb meets the metacarpal bone of the wrist. The reason this problem is so serious is that without a ligament to act as a kind of organic doorstop for the movement of the thumb, which allows you to impose leverage, your thumb would swing wide open, and you'd be unable to grip. The thumb is beyond doubt the most crucial digit on the hand—key to all the finer hand-to-eye coordination, and responsible for elevating us to the top of the evolutionary heap, besides.

This condition is also known as "gamekeeper's thumb," for the syndrome was first diagnosed in nineteenth century Scotland where gamekeepers snapped the necks of rabbits so often that they ruptured the thumb ligament. Left untreated, this particular problem can be quite serious. The smallest real injury, not merely to the thumb, but to the hand generally, can have a devastating impact on a person's life, particularly if that person is involved in a trade or art using manual dexterity: carpenters, visual artists, musicians, and so forth.

In skiing, the injury occurs when you fall with your ski pole handle between your thumb and index finger. I once gave myself a good tear at precisely this part of my hand, and being the macho idiot I am, decided to fix it myself (I was not yet a doctor at the time). My backwoods improvisation allowed me to keep skiing for the rest of the week, but also caused me a permanently painful condition. My only consolation is that I'm not alone: skiier's thumb is so pervasive that ski gloves are now designed with a malleable cast to protect you if you fall, and pole manufacturers likewise have come up with a variety of possible solutions.

Fractures

Being thin, and at the same time connected to the powerful muscles of the arms, the bones of the hand will occasionally suffer a full-blown fracture. Any obvious fracture should clearly be seen by an orthopedist as soon as possible. Fractures can be treated with a cast, and may sometimes need to be pinned for proper realignment. One of the most common fractures I see is what's called "the boxer's fracture," a characteristic break of the bone leading to the fifth metacarpal or pinkie, specifically. Almost invariably, it is caused by someone punching a wall—or a person. When people come to me with this complaint, I usually don't say anything at first, and let the patient concoct a half-baked story about how a can of beans fell on his hand, or the steam iron suddenly attacked her. Finally, at the right moment, I say: "so who did you punch?" Invariably, this brings a smile, and the truth.

Nailbed Injuries

Crushed hands tend to produce *hematomas*—blood that has pooled under the nailbed, and given you that faintly Transylvanian look. They are often associated with a fracture of the bone beneath the nail, a cut on the nailbed itself, or simply a powerful bruise—the classic case is that of a carelessly used hammer. The pressure of the blood is very painful, and in certain cases, permanent deformity can result. Nailbed injuries heal very slowly. They can also be drained by a physician, using the old pin-in-the-nail trick.

Now that you have an understanding of the anatomy of the hand and wrist and their most common injuries, let's continue on to Part One of the Bio-Point Exam.

The BIO-POINT Exam

Hand and Wrist

PART ONE

Question 1

Is there any deformity in the afflicted area? Look in the mirror and if possible compare the affected and the unaffected side. Is there a lack of symmetry?

If "yes," see a doctor immediately.

If "no," read on.

Question 2

Is there a severe limitation in your range of motion? Are you incapable of performing basic household tasks with the afflicted extremity?

If "yes," see a doctor immediately.

If "no," read on.

Question 3

Is there any sign of extensive or excessive swelling?

If "yes," see a doctor immediately.

If "no," read on.

Question 4

Are you afflicted with severe weakness in the injured body part? Do you have difficulty, for example, gripping a can?

If "yes," see a doctor immediately.

If "no," read on.

Question 5

Was a loud "pop" heard at the time of the injury?

If "yes," see a doctor immediately.

If "no," read on.

PART TWO

Whew! You're still with me! That's very good news because it means your injury may fall within the guidelines of what is treatable at home. What I'm going to do now is to zero in on your problem and attempt to make a more accurate diagnosis. Look at the accompanying illustration and touch the area where your pain or discomfort is most specific and localized. Note the number and the name of the injury (on the illustration) that corresponds with this area. Based on the

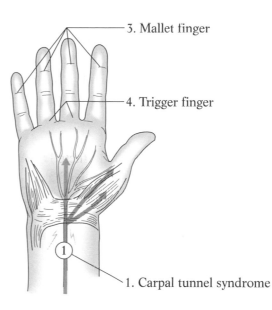

3. Mallet finger

4. Trigger finger

1. Carpal tunnel syndrome

area of pain you've indicated, this is likely to be the correct diagnosis. However, remember that injuries often overlap! Therefore, I recommend that you don't leap to any conclusion. Follow through by doing *all* of the

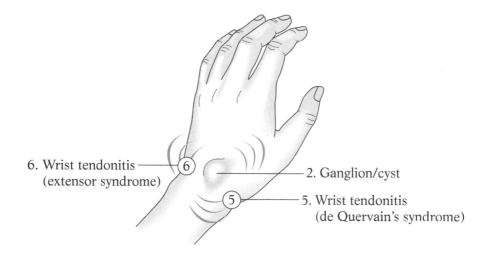

6. Wrist tendonitis (extensor syndrome)

2. Ganglion/cyst

5. Wrist tendonitis (de Quervain's syndrome)

Hand and Wrist • 73

Bio-Point Exams. This will ensure the most accurate and informed assessment of your injury. To help guide you in determining your own injury, each exam includes typical comments from patients suffering from that particular injury.

After each exam, the page number of the corresponding Med Unit is given. The Med Units are in Appendix A. Note: If no Med Unit is given, immediate medical attention is advised—since this condition cannot be treated at home. By following the Med Unit instructions, you can begin treating your injury immediately, keeping close track of your progress as you go.

1. Carpal Tunnel Syndrome

COMMENTS: "My hand is numb, especially my thumb and middle finger." "I wake up at night because of the pain." "There was no injury, it just suddenly began to hurt."

EXAM: Extend your arm outward with your palm facing up. Tap on the wrist crease in the very center. Do you feel shocks radiating down your hand and into your fingers?

THERAPY: See Med Unit, pages 169–170.

2. Ganglion/Cyst

COMMENTS: "I have a bump on my wrist."

EXAM: Gently probe the bump with your fingers. Is it soft and pliable? If so, it is most likely a ganglion.

THERAPY: See Med Unit, page 170.

3. Mallet Finger

COMMENTS: "I can't straighten my finger." (Often heard after playing football.)

EXAM: Extend your arm out straight in front of you—palm down. Attempt to straighten your fingers. Does the afflicted finger flop forward?

THERAPY: See a doctor who will most likely provide a splint. Most times this is not a problem that requires surgery.

4. Trigger Finger

COMMENTS: "My finger locks." "I can't open or close my finger." "There is a clicking in my finger."

EXAM: Open your palm facing you. Take the afflicted finger and move it in a clench toward the palm. Try to pull it back out again. Is there a locking or a clicking?

THERAPY: See Med Unit, page 170.

5. Wrist Tendonitis (de Quervain's Syndrome)

COMMENTS: "The base of my thumb hurts and I don't remember doing anything traumatic to it."

EXAM: Hold your hand palm side up. Put the thumb in the palm and curl the fingers around it (in a kind of fist). Now try to pull the fist outward from the base of the wrist. Is there pain on the outside of the wrist?

THERAPY: See Med Unit, page 170.

6. Wrist Tendonitis (Extensor Syndrome)

COMMENTS: "It hurts when I pull my hand back."

EXAM: Hold your hand in front of you, palm side down. Try to pull your hand back toward you against resistance. You can use your other hand to provide this resistance. Is there pain (particularly on the outside area of the wrist)?

THERAPY: See Med Unit, page 170.

7. Fractures and Sprains (Wrist and Hand)

COMMENTS: "I fell on my hand." "I can move my wrist and hand so it must not be fractured."

THERAPY: See a doctor immediately if you suspect you have a fractured wrist.

8. Sprains, Fractures, Dislocations (Fingers)

COMMENTS: "I jammed my finger." "My finger is crooked looking." "My thumb dislocated while I was skiing." "I can move my finger, so it must not be broken."

THERAPY: See a doctor immediately if any of these comments describes your condition.

6

Spine and Back

Back pain is an equal opportunity employer, and a workaholic to boot. Throbbing back pain attacks young as well as old, professional athletes as often as sedentary office workers, weekend warriors as easily as couch potatoes, and it attacks with amazing frequency. The phrase "My back hurts, Doc," sometimes seems to my ears like an orthopedic anthem of some kind, the medical equivalent of a hit single: twist and shout—my back is killing me!

When people say "back," of course, they include not only the long, fantastically intricate suspension bridge of the spine, but the vast overlapping fan of dorsal muscles that, together, constitute the most powerful muscular complex in the body. Graced with names like erector spinae, and trapezius, the intricate back muscles allow you the grace of walking upright, and not on all fours like our ancestors. However, this marvelous achievement comes with a price.

The fact is, we are a society of people with bad backs. At one time or another, upward of 90 percent of the American population will suffer from back pain. Back injuries are currently the leading occupational hazard in the U.S., with 25 million Americans claiming they lost at least a day's work from the pain and discomfort. Fortunately, traumatic back injuries are very rare in the kinds of sports most recreational athletes indulge in. More common are the garden-variety strains and sprains, which accrue on the playing fields and courts, and the soreness of overworked spinal columns. The back, in fact, gets sore so often, and so deeply at times, that one is tempted to ask: did God, in His infinite wisdom, pull an anatomical boner? Why should anything as structurally intrinsic to our lives as a back cause us such a world of pain?

The answer, of course, lies less with God and more with our sluggard habits.

We're too sedentary, too pampered physically, and too unaware of the vital functioning of our bodies. The spine is the place in the body where all the little oversights accumulate: we slump at work, we slouch when we stand, we sleep scrunched up. We weigh too much. With no stretching at all, we lie down and rattle off a hundred abdominal crunches—which can cause the spinal bones to chafe against one another like we're grinding coffee beans with our vertabrae. We carry a heavy weight without understanding the basic principles of leverage. We bend over too quickly, or on the tennis or golf or paddle tennis court whip those forehands, drives, and backhands into the far distance without ever paying any attention to the place that generates all the power: the back. The back is like the foot in that, being invisible for the most part, it is easy to ignore.

Sleep

The famous slogan we all grow up hearing runs, "You are what you eat." As far as the back is concerned, I'd revise that to, "You are how you sleep." Those eight hours a night you pass in dreamland have a key bearing on spinal health. First things first: choose a firm mattress, the firmer the better. Half the world sleeps on a hard floor, and we could learn something from their minimal arrangements. In the great Futon versus boxspring debate, I tend toward the boxspring. Futons are fine at first, but they fairly quickly lose their loft as they grow compressed from body weight. My own experience sleeping on one in college was that backaches soon followed. As for sleeping posture, the verdict is pretty cut and dry: sleeping on the stomach is not good for the back, and neither, surprisingly, is sleeping on the back itself. The best posture is on the side, in the fetal position, with the legs drawn up toward the chest—a position that provides relief for the lower back. It is best to try consciously to alternate sides from time to time, the better to equally distribute the stresses.

Driving

The automobile has not been especially friendly to backs. The combination of an upright driving position with the legs extended for long perids of time can produce real stress in the lower back, particularly when combined with the inevitable aggravation of traffic. One of the secrets of the raked sports-car seating position was that it allowed the body to relax, and took the stress off the vulnerable lumbar vertabrae. Car manufacturers have finally understood that the interior of a car is not only a visual but a biomechanical experience, and have begun making revisions in the classic "church pew" bench seat, the better to accomodate back fatigue. When driving, do your best not to slouch and effectively "sit" on your lower back. Make certain that your lower back is in contact with the lumbar portion of the seat. Try to find a seat that supports you rather than enveloping you in a soft, touchy-feely experience. If you have cruise control, set it on, retract your feet from the pedals and very carefully stretch upward in your seat. Do not drive for more than an hour or two without stopping to stretch your back.

Lifting

The key when fighting gravity with heavy objects is to use the muscles of the legs—the calves and thighs. Do not bend far forward using your back when lifting. Instead, always crouch using your quads and glutes. Think leverage at all times. Attempt con-

ANATOMY

Many people think of the spine as straight, but the spine is shaped with the lovely s-curve of a violin, or a sea horse. This curving structure allows the spine to expand and contract as necessary, while carrying the enormous weights and shearing stresses of a body in motion. Imagine a computer that is daily drop-kicked, sat on, and sideswiped, while continuing to process and feed back the data necessary to keep 100 planes airborne in perfect formation, and you'll have the beginnings—the barest beginnings—of an idea of what the spine does.

The spine begins at the very top of the neck, just below the occipital lobe of the brain, where an extension of the brain called the brain stem is located. Of the twenty-six total vertebrae in the back, seven are right there, in the neck or cervical region, holding up the thick casing of the skull and the wonder-custard of the brain itself. How thick is the skull case? So thick that the average NHL forward, to take a particularly violent example, can have his head whanged into the boards a thousand times in his career, and walk away from it with his pension, his faculties, and his double vision intact.

Below the cervical vertabrae are the twelve thoracic vertabrae, which support the ribs, and is commonly known as the midback. Situated below these, in turn, are the lumbar vertabrae, which can be said to be the heavy lifters, the workhorses of the spine (Fig. 6.1). It is the fate of

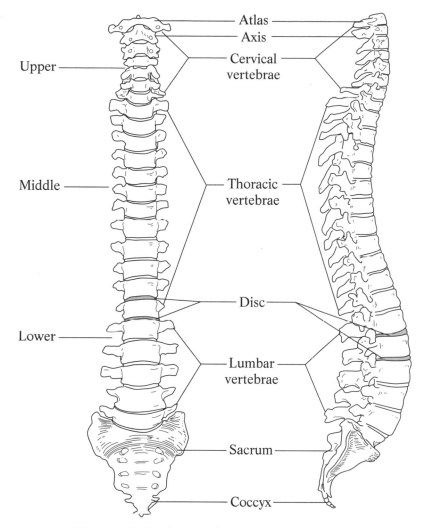

Upper

Middle

Lower

Atlas
Axis
Cervical
vertebrae
Thoracic
vertebrae
Disc
Lumbar
vertebrae
Sacrum
Coccyx

Fig. 6.1 (Left): front and (right): side views of the spine.

these lowest five spinal knobs to suffer the worst mechanical strains and stresses of the entire skeletal structure. Nothing else in the body works so hard and receives so little attention. Constantly under stress, the lumbar vertebrae can truly be said to be the base of the upper body—chest, arms, and head: the bottom of the pyramid on top of which the upper torso stands. The lumbar spine is the most common area of complaint for back sufferers, the most commonly operated on place in the back—and, as mentioned, the thickest and heaviest of the vertabrae.

But not only the lumbar vertabrae are tough customers. All the spinal vertabrae are composed of very thick, durable material, and are built on the same principle of construction as the skull itself: with the hardest substance—bone—on the outside, and successively more delicate materials as you move toward the core of the spinal cord.

The Spinal Cord

The spinal cord looks deceptively modest to the naked eye—a strand of cut-rate twine or bloated spaghetti, but that cord is the actual superhighway along which all the nervous impulses that make the entity called Frank, or Jane, or in my case Andrew, are routed. Although it weighs only an ounce or so, and measures a mere 17 inches of length, it forks out into thirty-one nerves, which in their turn fork and fork again until they've covered the entire body with pure neural conductivity. The spinal cord is the anatomical equivalent of those old-fashioned switchboards from the screwball comedies in which busy operators were always frantically plugging and pulling phone wires to make their connection. The difference is that the operators dialing in your spine take no vacations and never sleep! Their work is hampered by the many things that can dampen the neurological dial tone—a disc pressing on a nerve or cord, a hollowing of the canal, or arthritis, to name three. Any of these factors can precipitate an inflammatory response that will interfere with the strength and clarity of the signal being transmitted by the nerve. And if the signal is compromised, pain, weakness, numbness, and even paralysis will follow.

As a way of cushioning the shocks of life and preventing this kind of impingement, your spine incorporate, a system of floating shock absorbers or pads, which lie between the vertabrae to soften the stresses. These are the infamous

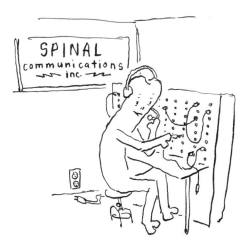

"Yes, I'd like to be connected to the lobe for pain-free wealth, please."

discs, which are actually tough little compartments of gristle filled with a gel called *nucleosus pulposus*. Imagine, instead of a spine, a stack of peanut butter and jelly sandwiches. When compressed or overly stressed, the contents of those sandwiches will bulge. In the case of the spine, that bulging gel is what we call a *slipped disc* (Fig. 6.2). Nothing has actually slipped, per se. Rather, the walls of the disc, under tremendous pressure, have begun to bulge—and that bulge or rupture impinges on the spinal nerves, causing a characteristic pain and weakness. When torn, the disc will spill its gel into the spinal column, where it will harden against the nerves, creating intense pain and requiring immediate surgery.

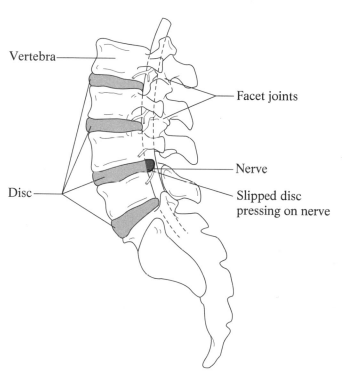

Fig. 6.2 Lumbar spine (lower back) with slipped disc.

The good news for anyone suffering from slipped or bulging discs is that the commoness of the bad back has forced an explosion of research into noninvasive procedures for repairing slipped discs and spinal problems generally. Once, for example, the spinal fusion was fairly common—a last-ditch procedure in which a ground powder of bone and glue was used somewhat like a tire patch to fill the hole left by a blown disc, thereby rendering the back much less flexible in the process. Now there are a variety of microscopic disc surgeries involving much less invasive means than previously. Eventually, doctors may be able to selectively dissolve tissue with an injection, rendering certain kinds of spinal surgery entirely obsolete.

One of the things driving this kind of research, and medical research generally, is the perfect anatomical consistency of the body. Cell by cell, limb by limb, system by system, bodies are uniformly the same, allowing for variation in size. A collossal road map has been drawn by God, and through years of testing, doctors have learned their way down not merely the main thoroughfares, but the shady lanes and alleys as well. Nowhere is this more true than in the spine, whose precious cargo of nerves is both fantastically complex, and is also on the brink of giving up its secrets. The regeneration of spinal cord nerves is *THE* issue currently on the boards in a lot of neurological research. If the past is any indication, we're not that far away from cracking its code.

INJURIES

Back health is influenced by a variety of factors. Some of the most important ones are overall fitness and tone. Cardiovascular fitness, for example, helps maintain the bone mass that is so important to a healthy spine. Also important are the limberness of the hamstrings and the hip-flexor joints, and the tone of the abdominal muscles, whose appearance of a brick wall (when healthy) should remind you that they are in fact a structural brace for the spinal column. Occupational hazards can be a factor too, as those with certain kinds of jobs involving repeated bending and lifting can often suffer from overuse injuries to the back.

With its musculoskeletal complexity, its central nature to all sports and the manifold stresses it undergoes, the back is of course prey to a wide variety of aches and pains. The majority of these, as mentioned, are lumbosacral (the sacrum is the bony plate at the very bottom of the back, a kind of stabilizer bar for the spine rising above it). By and large, these are not serious problems, and don't require surgery. Yet these pains are often the hardest to get rid of. Why? Because they're usually based on lifestyle and learned behavior. Sometimes they're the fault of a specific twisting motion or an injury. But more likely they're related to stress, posture, alignment, and general fitness. A lot of people, from this point of view, are accidents waiting to happen. Too often they set themselves up subclinically by ignoring the normal care and maintenance of the back, pop up out of a ten-year slouch and go directly to the tennis court or weight room to rattle off some wicked strokes or lifts. The payoff for this is often a lovely week or two spent flat on one's back in bed, gobbling aspirin and hating daytime television.

SPECIFIC INJURIES

Ligament Strain

This is often the result of improper lifting, or of a sudden, unexpected rotation in a sporting event. Typically, a ligament strain announces itself with a sharp pain that deepens and intensifies in the next couple of hours. There are two dangers with ligament strains of the back. If they are serious enough, they can undermine the stability of the spinal column, and if not rehabilitated completely, they can predispose the spine to reinjure itself at the very same spot. A rough diagnostic tip: in the aftermath of a strain, localized pain is expected and appropriate. However if the pain begins to travel at all, seek immediate medical attention, because that generally indicates a compromised nerve.

Sciatica

This is an inflammation of the long, critical sciatic nerve, which runs from the lower back, through the hip joint, and down the leg. Sciatica is usually indicated by a characteristic numbness, weakness, and pain pattern. It does not require emergency medical treatment, but can become disabling if left alone and allowed to worsen, so you should seek medical attention.

Spondylosis

A stress fracture of the lower back to which gymnasts and young football players are prone, in which the lower back structures grow weak, begin to disintegrate, sometimes slide and overlap. Treatment often includes a brace, change of activity, or even surgery.

The Cervical Spine

The cervical or neck spine, though it mimicks its big brother the lumbar spine, is far more delicate and prone to serious injury. Part of the reason for this is that the neck spine is constructed for maximum swiveling mobility of the head, and with that mobility, as we now know, comes a price. The proximity of the neck to the skull means that injuries to the c-spine, as it's known, can also entail collateral injury to the cranium or brain. Leaving aside the ghastly scenario of the broken neck, the most common neck injuries are simple strains and sprains.

Neck Sprains and Strains

Like any muscular or ligamentous structure, the neck, when strained or sprained through trauma, produces very painful results. Whiplash anyone? One particular reason why neck trauma is so unbelievably painful is that the neck muscles, when traumatized, tend to lock rigid, the better to protect the area. Doctors often attempt to produce the same result with a neck brace, which likewise holds the neck immobile. Patience is required for neck sprains and strains, which take anywhere from five days to three weeks to heal.

Cervical "Stingers"

These pesky little tantrums of the cervical nerve are well known to athletes who participate in violent sports like football and rugby. A burning flash of pain down the side of the neck and arm, a cervical stinger is caused by the stretching of the cervical nerve. This is not of great concern if it happens only once in a while, as it does to most peope, but if it occurs often, it can cause bleeding and a buildup of scar tissue around the nerve, which will become disabling if left untreated by physical therapy including neck-strengthening exercises.

BACK PAIN TREATMENT

Any condition as prevalent, paralyzing, and painful as back distress will have a hundred different remedies and cures. These range from the crackpot to the credible, with a hundred variations in between. Two of the most popular are chiropractic and yoga, and though I think that chiropractic has its place, I tend to be wary of the promises and the pain relief it affords you.

The point of the matter is that your back is the way it is today because of all the many years you've lived in it, leaning on it, stretching with it, and feeling it tighten when your tax returns are due. It's a cumulative process, a learned process. A chiropractor may reach in and with a good crack temporarily relieve the pressure—which is no small feat, if there's pain involved—but the body will soon reassert itself, and return to its old habits.

Yoga is different because it's gradual, and also because YOU do the work, rather than having it passively done to you. It's an active, participatory way to change old habits. A good example of yoga positively influencing a life is that of Kareem Abdul Jabbar, the basketball great. In the days before the clinical importance of stretching was understood the way it is today, Abdul-Jabbar practiced yoga assiduously, a fact that enabled him to play with a relative lack of injury late into his thirties.

Saudi arms merchant Adnan Khashoggi was said to have a servant whose sole responsibility was to follow behind him and every twenty minutes give his neck a good crack. If nothing else, credit the Arab billionaire with understanding the transitory nature of chiropractic.

If you're not up to the particular tractions and contortions of yoga, try simple stretching. Appendix B contains basic back stretches, which can be found on pages 186–188. These work, and will provide relief.

Now that you have an understanding of the anatomy of the back and spine and their most common injuries, let's continue on to Part One of the Bio-Point Exam.

The BIO-POINT Exam

Spine and Back

PART ONE

Question 1

Is there any deformity in the afflicted area? Look in the mirror and if possible compare the affected and the unaffected side. Is there a lack of symmetry?
If "yes," see a doctor immediately.
If "no," read on.

Question 2

Is there a severe limitation in your range of motion? Are you incapable of performing basic household tasks with the afflicted extremity?
If "yes," see a doctor immediately.
If "no," read on.

Question 3

Is there any sign of extensive or excessive swelling?
If "yes," see a doctor immediately.
If "no," read on.

Question 4

Are you afflicted with severe weakness in the injured body part? Do you have difficulty, for example, climbing stairs?
If "yes," see a doctor immediately.
If "no," read on.

Question 5

Was a loud "pop" heard at the time of the injury?
If "yes," see a doctor immediately.
If "no," read on.

PART TWO

Whew! You're still with me! That's very good news because it means your injury may fall within the guidelines of what is treatable at home. What I'm going to do now is to zero in on your problem and attempt to make a more accurate diagnosis. Look at the accompanying illustration and touch the area where your pain or discomfort is most specific and localized. Note the number and the name of the injury (on the illustration) that corresponds with this area. Based on the area of pain you've indicated, this is likely to be the correct diagnosis. However, remember that injuries often overlap! Therefore, I recommend that you don't leap to any conclusions. Follow through by doing *all* of the Bio-Point Exams. This will ensure the most accurate and informed assessment of your injury. To help guide you in determining your own injury, each exam includes typical comments from patients suffering from that particular injury.

After each exam, the page number of the corresponding Med Unit is given. The Med Units are in Appendix A. Note: If no Med Unit is given, immediate medical attention is advised—since the condition cannot be treated at home. By following the Med Unit instructions, you can begin treating your injury immediately, keeping close track of your progress as you go.

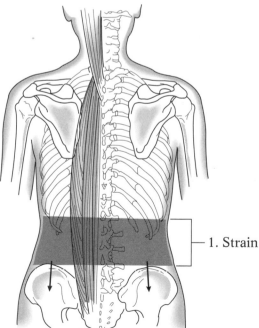

1. Strain

1. Low Back Strain:

COMMENTS: "My lower back feels tight." "I have localized pain in my back."

EXAM: As befits something of the complexity of the back, back strains come in all shapes and sizes, from a small pinging overworked muscle deep within the back to an agonizing rip. Tightness in the back without pain radiating down the buttock or leg tends to indicate a localized condition, without the more serious secondary consequences. This is treatable on your own. However, if the pain radiates, or is so severe that it frightens you, you should see a doctor immediately.

THERAPY: See Med Unit, page 171.

2. "Slipped" (Herniated) Disc/Sciatica

COMMENTS: "I have pains in my buttock, traveling down my leg." "I have numbness in my leg/foot." "My leg feels suddenly weak, for no reason."

EXAM: Lie on a bed, raise your leg, and flex your toes toward your head. Does that recreate the radiating symptoms from your back down your leg?

THERAPY: Slipped discs are very serious, and if you have any doubt at all about the condition, you should see a doctor immediately.

7

Knee

When skiing, one dreams of one thing above all: a cleansing fall of fresh snow. One travels great distances to find it. So you can imagine my joy several years ago during a vacation at Snowbird, in Utah, to find the flakes falling with the thickness and rapidity of lies from a campaigning politician. It was the very beginning of ski season, and I was itching to get out and begin carving turns. Unfortunately for me, the snowfall was so dense that for three days they had to close the slopes. During this time I developed a galloping case of what is called "lodge lock," a special kind of Rocky Mountain cabin fever, in which you sit very still, watch CNN for hours at a time, and observe the snow falling outside while feeling sudden strange affinities with the likes of Timothy Mcveigh. When they finally let us onto the slopes, I was impatient to get up and get skiing. Powder skiing is an entirely different experience from rushing downhill on hard-pack snow. One floats down the slope, nearly airborne. It's the closest thing to flying on land you can experience. Unfortunately for me, things didn't quite work out according to plan. Not long into my first run of the morning, I felt an edge catch, my skis cartwheel over my head, and plunge deep into the heavy snow. There was that doomed fraction of a second, during which I knew that I had a made a very, very large mistake. This was followed by the characteristic "pop." I had suffered a partial tear of the *medial collateral ligament*—an injury that bedevils football running backs and hockey players as well. A cheerful ski patrolman brought me down the hill in a bucket. I was out of commission for almost three months.

On the arthroscope, the knee doesn't look like much. An underwater cave scene from *Jacques Cousteau,* perhaps, filled with shadows and waving sea anemones. But in that cave lies the body's largest joint, an evolutionary curiosity whose biomechanics have fascinated doctors for centuries.

Part of this fascination derives from the fact that, from a load-bearing point of view, the knee is a miraculous construction. Built like the elbow as a simple hinge joint, the knee carries the awesome responsibility of holding the body upright during walking, running, and standing.

With that awesome responsibility comes a certain distinction: injury. The knee is the most injured joint in the body—more often injured than the elbow, the shoulder, or even the oft-twisted ankle. Why? Because of two main reasons, separated by a few million years: the boom in athletics over the last two decades, and the internal structure of the knee, which is the product of eons of evolution. You see, structurally the knee is quite weak. Despite its size and critical anatomical function, it is made out of delicate plates of cartilage surrounded by a mass of powerful leg muscles, which place the knee under incredible stresses, particularly during athletic events. Remember, as a hinge joint, the knee opens and shuts mainly in one direction. Great if you're in a parade, but less advantageous during athletic events, most of which contain plenty of the violent twisting motions and lateral movements that land knees in so much trouble. The knee can accommodate some side-to-side and rotational movement, but not much. And let's face it, nearly every sport contains enough of a rhumba to put the knee in trouble: touch football, the tennis backhand, the drive in golf—all the twisting stresses produced by these actions travel right up the omnidirectional ball and socket of the ankle, and lodge—where else— in the unprotected intersection of the knee.

So they complain, do our knees. In the last few years, orthopedic surgeons have witnessed huge increases in both overuse and traumatic injuries to the knee. The knee tendons snap with the characteristic "ping!" of a guitar string popping. Their mating surfaces roughen. Their cartilage wears away. They get arthritic, inflamed, and nearly useless. In certain cases, the knee can actually begin to die.

When healthy, the knee on the arthroscope screen appears pristine, with sharp rounded edges meeting in perfect alignment and stability. But when suffering overuse injuries or trauma, this same knee takes on the look of shredded clothes, with dribs and drabs of cartilage hanging everywhere. This cartilage-confetti doesn't heal naturally, because the knee joint works in a lubricating bath of specialized fluid, and is without blood supply. The reason I know so much about the look of knees is because I've worked on so many of them over the years. They're one of my surgical specialties. I've helped pioneer treatment techniques. In addition to this, of course, there was my own busted knee.

ANATOMY

The joint I injured that snowy day while skiing has a very basic function: to broker the stresses of locomotion. For the most part, it performs this task superbly, but it's easily hurt. The reasons for this, as usual, can be found in the anatomy. From an anatomical point of view, the knee is simply the meeting place of the upper leg bone or femur, and the lower leg

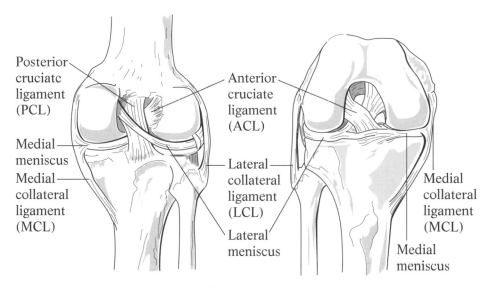

Fig. 7.1 (Left): back and (right): front views of the knee.

bone, or tibia. To keep this crucial joint stable, nature worked a bit overtime and came up with an ingenious system. You've heard of the Cross Your Heart bra? The knee has cross-your-heart ligaments, and some other wonderfully unique shock-absorption technology built right in. First, the knee is stabilized by two entirely different ligamentous systems. One forms the sleevelike connection between the two large leg bones, and is called the knee capsule. Ligaments run through this sheath, a bit like the metal plies of a radial tire, to strengthen it. These capsule ligaments, which are called the medial collateral (MCL) and the lateral collateral (LCL) ligaments, provide much of the hinging action and the extension of the knee. But because the knee takes side-to-side stress, too, nature wisely provided two internal crossing ligaments, called the cruciate ligaments—the anterior cruciate (ACL), which crosses in the front, and the posterior cruciate (PCL), which crosses in the back (Fig 7.1).

The meeting place of these two large leg bones is crucial, so not only are there these various fantastically engineered ligament systems there to oversee a happy outcome, but the heads of the bones are notched to fit one into the other. The knobs on the ends of the thighbones or femurs—a chicken bone has these too—are called condyles. The bones sit in crescent-shaped pads of specialized cartilage on the tops of the tibia called meniscus cartilage. These meniscus pads are on the firing line of the stress of walking and running, and to keep from being ground to talcum powder, are bathed in a constant flow of lubricating solution from the bursa, the small pouches that are scattered through the joints of the body like tiny oil pumps, providing crucial slipperiness at the mating surfaces. Meniscal cartilage is highly specialized, and distinct from the rest of the cartilage in the body. The kneecap itself, or patella, is the thick front door that protects all the delicate engineering behind it.

INJURIES

As with most other joints, injuries to the knee break down into the groupings of *chronic* and *acute*. Almost all acute knee injuries involve the same biomechanical snafu: the foot is planted and the leg is either then torqued or twisted, alone, with the help of a piece of a equipment like a ski, or your friendly neighborhood nose tackle. Obviously, my skiing injury was as acute as it gets: a rip of the medial collateral ligament. This injury is first cousin to **ACL injuries,** which are perhaps the most common of all traumatic knee ligament injuries. Roughly 60 percent of all serious knee ligament injuries involve damage to this piece of fibrous tissue. When a 360-pound lineman by the name of "Train" makes chicken bones out of a quarterback's legs, yanking them as if to break away the wishbones, he often begets an ACL tear. The little letters ACL strike fear into even the bravest professional athlete, because they almost invariably spell DL (disabled list). The ligament itself is a tough, multiply stranded cord, which will only give up and tear completely after a real fight.

You should remember that most ligament sprains will heal on their own, and that they rarely require surgery. Instead, careful placing, bracing, and physical therapy can get the ligaments to knit back to their original condition. The healing rate of knee sprains is directly dependent on the severity of trauma suffered by that particular ligament. Sprains to the ligaments of the knee are graded level I, II, or III. A grade I sprain is fairly minor, and usually will have you out of athletics for a week or so. A grade II injury will cost in the neighborhood of three weeks to heal. A grade III, which is what I suffered on the snowy slopes that day, is is a

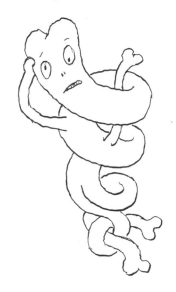

"Come on baby let's do the twist. Come on baby let's rip our knees like this."

complete tear that need to be operated on to stitch the knee back together.

An ACL injury can be treated conservatively, but it sometimes leads athletes afflicted with it to give up their sport entirely, particularly if that sport involves many of the twisting motions that landed them in hot water in the first place. ACL surgery was only formerly done on young athletes, but the boom in recreational athletics and the subsequent rise of golden-oldie weekend warriors (along with the increasing noninvasiveness of the surgery itself) has led to it having a much wider application than could have previously been imagined.

Another fairly common injury to the knee is a **tear in the meniscal cartilage**. This can happen acutely, through a torquing incident in which a piece of the cartilage is wrenched away from its mooring, or chronically, through wear and tear. To my patients I often liken meniscus wear to the beloved shirt that, after one hundred washings, fades and then, on that fatal day, tears clean through. Like that shirt, the meniscus cannot repair itself, and must be shaved clean with an arthoscope, in the classic bread and butter knee surgery of an orthopedic surgeon. This condition typically announces itself with a clicking and locking—as if someone jammed a wedge in the door of your stride.

Did you think that was all? Not by a long shot! The specialized articular cartilage on the ends of the bones that terminate at the knee can also be damaged, both acutely, and more commonly, through routine wear and tear. For all intents and purposes, this is **arthritis of the knee**. It has the same inflammatory response as arthritis, and like arthritis, is difficult to treat, because it is a progressive degenerative problem. Common treatment regimens include: weight reduction, braces, icing, lessening the impact load, and as a last resort, an arthroscopic "spring cleaning" of the knee. Unfortunately, even surgery doesn't guarantee complete relief.

OTHER KNEE INJURIES

Patella-Femoral Syndrome

This mouthful (sometimes known by an even more indigestible mouthful, "chondromalacia") describes a syndrome that is very common to runners, in which an inflammation develops on the underside of the knee. The kneecap has somehow becomes misaligned in its groove, and begins to slip out and rub on the sides of the groove, causing the cartilage under the knee to wear out, and fluid to occasionally build up and cause swelling in the knee. About 20 percent of my patients with knee problems suffer from this. It can derive from the structural fact of a badly "built" knee, from the dynamic fact of a muscle imbalance (in which case physical therapy can help), or by the mechanical fact of sheer overuse in athletics. The onset is gradual, and patients typically report the sensation of a toothache in the knee, accompanied by a grinding and popping. Sitting for extended periods, climbing stairs (or StairMasters), and step classes can all aggravate the condition. It is common in women, whose wider hips and turned-in knees predispose

A Tip on Muscle Imbalance

A key to remember with chronic-use knee difficulties is that they are often caused by muscle imbalance. This imbalance can be corrected with specific exercise to strengthen the quadriceps, the four large interlaced thigh muscles, which allow you to generate much of the force of your forward motion. On the other hand, if overworked, or worked incorrectly, these big muscles can produce a tendonitis at the knee attachment. Both this, and the imbalance that can cause other, more serious knee problems, can be corrected with simple exercise and physical therapy.

them toward it. Eighty to 90 percent of patients get better with treatment, and don't require surgery.

Osteochondritis Dissecans

This terrifying sounding condition forms when the ends of the leg bones, grinding against one another, eventually dislodge a bit of their superslick mating surface. The injury resembles a divot dug with a golf club. In time, this piece grows loose and begins to cause pain. The dissecans in the name of this syndrome refers to a dissection of a loose piece from the surface of the joint. If the piece falls free, it's like a stick in the spokes of a bicycle—jamming the knee frozen. Sometimes the piece actually begins to migrate through the knee. It is called "joint mice" because it is white and skitters around the knee. Most of the time surgery is necessary.

Iliotibial Band Inflammation

This is an overuse syndrome, which is as common as rain to runners, mainly of longer distances. In this situation, the iliotibial band of fibrous

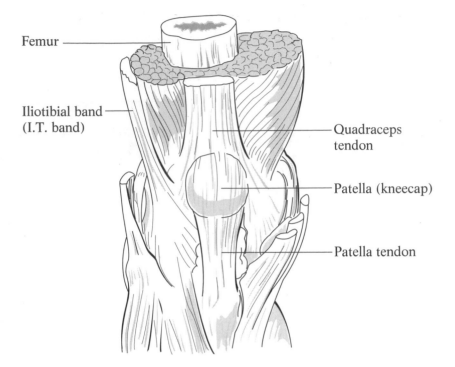

Femur

Iliotibial band
(I.T. band)

Quadraceps
tendon

Patella (kneecap)

Patella tendon

Fig. 7.2 Front view of knee.

tissue (see Fig. 7.2) which runs down the outer part of the thigh to the knee and acts as a lateral stabilizer of sorts for the leg and hip can cause difficulties if it grows too taut, or becomes inflamed from microtrauma. It is important to note that this most often produces a generalized pain, which is not specific but seems to be located in a broad area on the outer part of the joint. Typically, among runners, this condition will produce pain about 15 minutes into the run, and that pain will get progressively worse until they have to stop. When they cease running, the pain will go away, but will return about 15 minutes into the next run. The condition, in which the overly tight band saws against the knee and outer hip, is often worsened by irregularities in the step and gait. These in turn are usually the product of pronation or supination. A look at your running shoes can actually help determine this almost as categorically as a medical exam. If you're a supinator, meaning if you tend to land first on the outside of your feet and then roll in, the outer edges of your shoes wear down quickly, while the inner areas over the ball of the foot look relatively untouched. If you're a pronator, that is, if your ankles tend to roll in excessively when you walk or stand, then your shoes will be worn down on the inside of the sole. Both conditions are usually cured with specific stretches and some handy-dandy orthotics.

Broken Kneecap

Occasionally, due to a fall on a hard surface, the tough knob of bone known as the kneecap can fracture. This can be a little tricky to diagnose, because certain people have a kneecap that is naturally formed in two pieces, and can deceive, without an X ray. Depending on the nature of the break, the knee will either have to be immobilized or operated on.

Shin Splints

Shin splints is the classic label for a certain kind of pervasive irritation felt, naturally enough, along the shin. Usually occurring among distance runners, it is the result of the pounding of the leg against hard pavement. But the term shin splints is really a catchall term, which embraces a variety of different lower-leg conditions. The pain formerly lumped under shin splints may in fact be: *periostitis* (inflamation of the covering of the tibia), *compartment syndrome* (swelling of the muscles of the leg within their individual membranous "compartments" in such a way that pain and discomfort results), or *stress fractures* of the tibia and fibula. The symptoms of these conditions are felt in different and specific places: pain behind the leg, on the upper calf, is usually posterior compartment syndrome. When felt on the front lower leg, it is usually anterior compartment syndrome, or stress fracture. On the outer side of the lower leg, usually later compartment syndrome or stress fracture. On the inner side of the lower leg, the pain is usually the result of periostitis, with the tibia's covering inflamed. Most of these conditions can be remedied with changes in footwear, orthotics, cessation of activity, and anti-inflamatory medication, but it is important to get a correct diagnosis, because, left untreated, these conditions can become disabling, and even permanent.

Now that you have an understanding of the anatomy of the knee and its most common injuries, let's continue on to Part One of the Bio-Point Exam.

The BIO-POINT Exam

K n e e

PART ONE

Question 1
Is there any deformity in the afflicted area? Look in the mirror and if possible compare the affected and the unaffected side. Is there a lack of symmetry?
If "yes," see a doctor immediately.
If "no," read on.

Question 2
Is there a severe limitation in your range of motion? Are you incapable of performing basic household tasks with the afflicted extremity?
If "yes," see a doctor immediately.
If "no," read on.

Question 3
Is there any sign of extensive or excessive swelling?
If "yes," see a doctor immediately.
If "no," read on.

Question 4
Are you afflicted with severe weakness in the injured body part? Do you have difficulty, for example, climbing stairs?
If "yes," see a doctor immediately.
If "no," read on.

Question 5
Was a loud "pop" heard at the time of the injury?
If "yes," see a doctor immediately.
If "no," read on.

PART TWO

Whew! You're still with me! That's very good news because it means your injury may fall within the guidelines of what is treatable at home. What I'm going to do now is to zero in on your problem and attempt to make a more accurate diagnosis. Look at the accompanying illustration and touch the area where your pain or discomfort is most specific and localized. Note the number and the name of the injury (on the illustration) that corresponds with this area. Based on the area of pain you've indicated, this is likely to be the correct diagnosis. However, remember that injuries often overlap! Therefore, I recommend that you don't leap to any conclusion. Follow through by doing *all* of the Bio-Point Exams. This will

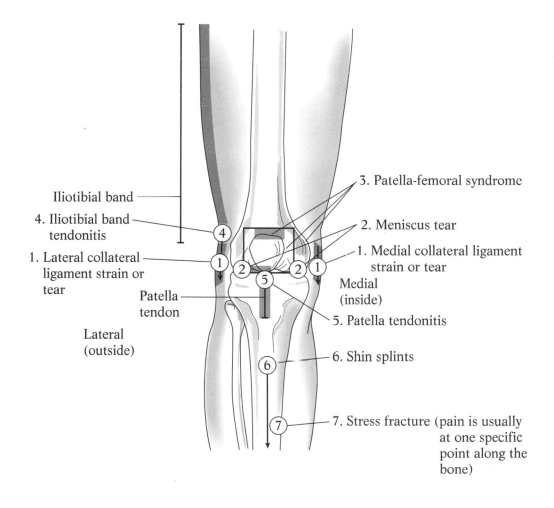

Iliotibial band

4. Iliotibial band tendonitis

1. Lateral collateral ligament strain or tear

Patella tendon

Lateral (outside)

3. Patella-femoral syndrome

2. Meniscus tear

1. Medial collateral ligament strain or tear

Medial (inside)

5. Patella tendonitis

6. Shin splints

7. Stress fracture (pain is usually at one specific point along the bone)

ensure the most accurate and informed assessment of your injury. To help guide you in determining your own injury, each exam includes typical comments from patients suffering from that particular injury.

After each exam, the page number of the corresponding Med Unit is given. The Med Units are in Appendix A. Note: If no Med Unit is given, immediate medical attention is advised—since the condition cannot be treated at home. By following the Med Unit instructions, you can begin treating your injury immediately, keeping close track of your progress as you go.

1. Medial/Lateral Collateral Ligament Strain or Tear

COMMENTS: "I twisted my knee." "It hurts on the inside/outside of my knee."

EXAM: Is there swelling? Is the knee black and blue? Is there a feeling of instability on either the inner or outer side of the knee? If so, see a doctor right away. If not, proceed to "therapy."

OTHER COMMENTS: This injury is typically seen among football players, skiiers, and snowboarders.

THERAPY: If pain is minimal and there is no feeling of instability, proceed to Med Unit, page 171.

2. Meniscus Tear

COMMENTS: "I twisted my knee. It seemed to recover but I still can't do everything I did before." "My knee is locking up."

EXAM: While flexing or extending the knee, probe with a finger at the inner and outer joint of the knee . Is there pain?

OTHER COMMENTS: If the injury is the result of a trauma or if the pain is severe, see a doctor. Otherwise, proceed to "therapy." This injury is commonly seen in sports that rely heavily on constant torque of the knee such as basketball, football, tennis, and skiing.

THERAPY: see Med Unit, pages 171–172.

3. Patella-Femoral Syndrome

COMMENTS: "It hurts when I take stairs." "I can no longer use the Stair-Master." "I have trouble squatting or sitting."

EXAM: Try to press your fingers underneath the kneecap. Is there pain? Go up and down the stairs. Try to stand and squat. Is there pain under the kneecap or in the knee?

THERAPY: See Med Unit, page 172.

4. Iliotibial Band Tendonitis

COMMENTS: "I feel pain and burning in my outer knee, usually when running and specifically on hills."

EXAM: Press on the area indicated on the illustration. Is there pain? Does the pain worsen with exertion, specifically running?

THERAPY: See Med Unit, page 172.

5. Patella Tendonitis

COMMENTS: "The front of my knee hurts when I land from jumping."

EXAM: Press over the area indicated on the illustration. Is there a sharp, specific pain? Now, jump in the air and come down as hard as you can tolerate. Is there pain in the area when landing? Does the pain worsen with jumping sports generally?

THERAPY: See Med Unit, pages 172–173.

6. Shin Splints

COMMENTS: "I have pain up and down my shin when I run, mostly on the inside of my leg."

EXAM: Ask yourself, is there generalized tenderness on the inner part of the bone of the lower leg? Now sit with your legs out in front of you and bend your feet inward against resistance (you may need someone to provide resistance). Does this either cause or worsen a generalized pain along the inner part of the shin?

THERAPY: See Med Unit, page 173.

7. Stress Fracture

COMMENTS: "I have a point of intense pain in my shin."

EXAM: Ask yourself, am I experiencing a specific, localized pain in my shin, not generalized as in shin splints? Is there specific tenderness along the inner part of the leg? Now, sit with you legs out in front of you, raise your leg and tap your heel with your knuckles (you may need someone to tap your heel for you.) Does a pain radiate to the area along the shin?

THERAPY: See a doctor.

8. Osteochondritis Dissecans

COMMENTS: "I feel a locking or clicking in my knee."

EXAM: Flex and extend your knee. Is there extensive popping or catching in the knee? Is there swelling of the knee that has not resolved itself?

THERAPY: See a doctor.

9. ACL Tear (Anterior Cruciate Ligament Tear)

COMMENTS: "I heard a loud pop." "My knee shifted." "My knee when out suddenly."

EXAM: Does your knee look swollen and feel "loose."

THERAPY: An ACL tear is an almost impossible injury to determine on your own. See a doctor right away.

8

Foot

Humblest of servants, buckled into boots, mashed into the toe-torturing triangles of high heels, the foot is mummified in heavy socks and left alone until pain or an odor like something dying awakens us to its presence. And yet the foot is the foundation stone of the skeleton, its root and base. When things go wrong with this limb, they rarely limit themselves exclusively to the foot itself but spread themselves upward thought the body in an "injury cascade": a rainbow of joint, tendon, and muscular ailments.

We rarely look at our feet from closer than five or six feet away, and yet, in terms of bones per square inch, the foot is probably the most complicated body part south of the hips, a pair of miniaturized spines whose load-bearing powers are staggering. Take the basic math of it: the average mile has 1,800 steps to it, and the average person walks four miles a week. Thirty-two thousand times a week, in other words, that foot is asked to absorb the downward pressure of the entire body weight, and then push off. Remember how you're always told to roll when you fall? Well the foot must roll with the poundage of the downward stroke of each footstep, and then lock rigid a moment, to push off the weight. This skeletal cha-cha takes place every time you walk: a gyration of locking and unlocking. When you run, the entire profile of the foot changes radically, as the weight it is asked to bear takes a dramatic increase.

When running, you have a phase of your locomotion called the "float phase" during which both feet are off the ground. When the foot does touch the ground again there is a proportionate increase in the downward force of the strike. During running, the vertical forces increase to a total of three to four times body weight with each footstep. Obviously, if a runner is either overweight or has a malalignment syndrome, these forces can be multiplied further. And if the person, overweight or thin, is training for a distance running event, the amount of pounding that the poor foot has to absorb rapidly turns exponential.

Many of the major movements in athletic activity that seem to have nothing to do with the foot—in fact draw directly from this limb. When Evander Holyfield slammed Mike Tyson's chin from below with a savage uppercut, or Michael Jordan flew through the air like a great bird en route to slam-dunking a game-winner, they each relied heavily on the push, the absorption, and the bounce of the foot.

ANATOMY

The foot is composed of a cat's cradle of bones, muscles, and nerves—which is why, in spy films and westerns, the stomped foot is always such a great disabling method of attack. Twenty-six bones and thirty joints are

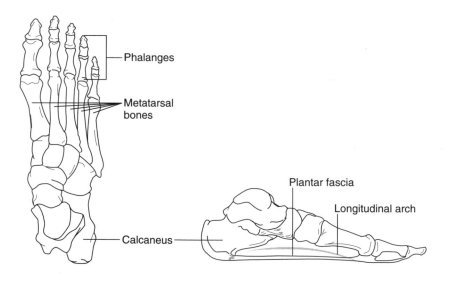

Fig. 8.1 (Left): top (dorsal) and (right): side views of the foot.

laid out in two arches, the longitudinal arch, leading from heel to toe, and the anterior arch, leading crosswise across the toes (Fig. 8.1). Both of these must flex in synchrony to absorb the weight of the footstrike, and stiffness or anatomical abnormalities in either can spell difficulties in sports.

In the same way that a bridge like the Golden Gate or the Brooklyn Bridge is not only beautiful, but, because of its arches, perfectly balanced to bear the billion-ton load of traffic, day in, and day out, so the arches of the foot have been arranged to support all of the muscles and ligaments of the legs and to bear the incredible weight of the body: walking, running, twisting, and turning (Figs 8.2 and 8.3). The foot is both durable and lightweight—if it were a piece of sporting gear, it would be one of

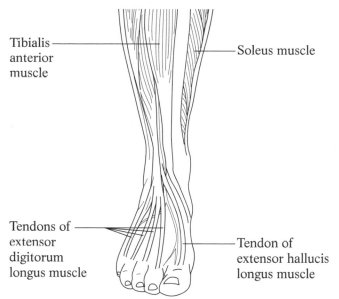

Fig. 8.2 Front view of the foot and leg.

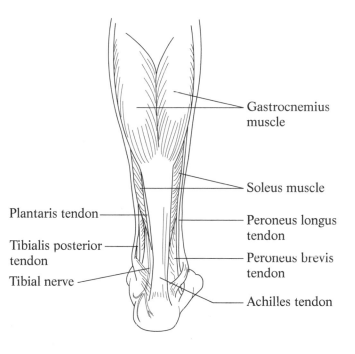

Fig. 8.3 Back view of the foot and leg.

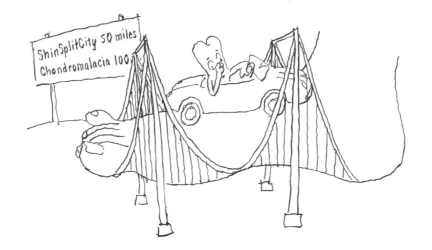

"Yes, the foot is an engineering marvel like a suspension bridge. But phew, don't they realize cartoons have a sense of smell?"

those beautifully engineered titanium bicycles, which convert the up-and-down driving power of the legs into forward motion. The foot does the same thing, but with far greater efficiency. Among the many design miracles of the body, the foot occupies a special place because of the disproportion between its small size and its load-bearing wizardry.

INJURIES

The foot is the initiator of your walk, the most characteristic human motion. As such, it has a role to play in nearly all pain involving the leg. Too often, when you have chronic hip or knee pain, you assume there is something wrong with those joints. In fact, anyone who has problems in their lower extremities, be they hip, or knee, shin or thigh, must first check the foot.

Because of its complexity, and the amount of nerves wound through it, the foot is full of small pinpoint areas, which, if irritated, can completely disable someone. The most minor inflammatory response or bone spur can affect a person's gait and stop him in his tracks.

Here are some typical foot problems:

Turf Toe

This is an inflammatory response that comes from stubbing your toe too many times against a nongiving surface like AstroTurf. This is a classic athletic injury, which happens as easily in basketball as football. If you're a "dragger" in tennis, dragging your foot when you serve, this is a common occurrence. A word on the pain of this injury: I've seen tough-as-nails 300-pound football players playing with broken noses and dislocated shoulders who are *immobilized* by the pain of turf toe, centered in a one-inch area under the big toe.

Metatarsalgia

A chronic garden-variety inflammation under the ball of the foot, metarsalgia is an overuse injury caused by malalignment, playing on bad surfaces, improper technique or the wrong footwear. For more information on footwear, please see Chapter 10 pages 132–133. In the meantime, remember, if your contact lenses are dirty or ripped, you get a new pair. Do the same with running and athletic shoes, too. As a general rule of thumb, you shouldn't wear a sneaker more than six months. If you're doing an activity like training for a marathon, the interval of shoe change should be even shorter.

Morton's Neuroma

Though this sounds like a kosher hors d'oeuvre, it is in fact a weedlike overgrowth of the nerve in the web spaces of the toes, which causes great pain. Typically this is described as a pain like an electric shock. It is often caused by too-narrow footwear. Not a tumor, it is a space-occupying lesion that causes pain as it grows. Usually it will resolve on its own. If not, a cortisone shot or the surgical removal of the neuroma may be necessary.

Sesamoiditis

This is an inflammatory response of the two floating bones under the ball of the big toe. These bones float in the same manner the patella does over the knee. Often ballet dancers who have to go on point suffer from this condition. These tiny bones can fragment under stress, and in so doing can end a dancer's career.

Plantar Fasciitis

This inflammatory condition is similar to tennis elbow in its commonness and its disabling effects. The longitudinal or plantar arch is the actual central structure of the foot. It mimics its big brother the spinal column by employing a curved array of joints to distribute the stresses, much like a suspension bridge. A thick, fibrous bundle of tissue called the plantar fascia is the "roadway" of this bridge, running the long way on the bottom of the foot and connecting the heel to the toes. When this fibrous bundle gets inflamed, it triggers the very common condition of plantar fasciitis, an injury syndrome that is the bread and butter of many an orthopedic surgeon. The hallmark of this condition is excessive pain in the arches when getting out of bed in the morning. As the day wears on, the pain usually subsides, but is exacerbated by excessive walking and sports. It is extremely difficult to deal with, for the simple reason that it is very hard to keep people off their feet. Their typical comment to me is: "The first couple steps kill me, Doc, but then it feels better." I explain to them that the danger in this condition, pain aside, is that if left untreated too long it will develop into a heel spur, an actual nodular growth at the site where the plantar fascia attaches to the heel. This is often so incapacitating that people can't walk. Classic causes for this are excess weight and the wrong footwear.

Stress Fracture

Repeated pounding causes microfractures of the bone, which cumulatively end up breaking the bone all the way through. This is usually seen in people who are doing repetitive, excessive athletic activity. Often called March Fractures, for their commonness among soldiers suddenly called upon to march long distances without any preparation, stress fractures are difficult to diagnose because they don't show up early on, are difficult to see on X-rays (at the onset), and can mimic problems like tendonitis and ligament strains. If you have persistent, unremitting pain, you should probably be seen by an orthopedic doctor, where a special *bone scan* or X-ray may be necessary.

Now that you have an understanding of the anatomy of the foot and its most common injuries, let's continue on to Part One of the Bio-Point Exam.

The BIO-POINT Exam

F o o t

PART ONE

Question 1
Is there any deformity in the afflicted area? Look in the mirror and if possible compare the affected and the unaffected side. Is there a lack of symmetry?
If "yes," see a doctor immediately.
If "no," read on.

Question 2
Is there a severe limitation in your range of motion? Are you incapable of performing basic household tasks with the afflicted extremity?
If "yes," see a doctor immediately.
If "no," read on.

Question 3
Is there any sign of extensive or excessive swelling?
If "yes," see a doctor immediately.
If "no," read on.

Question 4
Are you afflicted with severe weakness in the injured body part? Do you have difficulty, for example, climbing stairs?
If "yes," see a doctor immediately.
If "no," read on.

Question 5
Was a loud "pop" heard at the time of the injury?
If "yes," see a doctor immediately.
If "no," read on.

Whew! You're still with me! That's very good news because it means your injury may fall within the guidelines of what is treatable at home. What I'm going to do now is to zero in on your problem and attempt to make a more accurate diagnosis. Look at the accompanying illustration and touch the area where your pain or discomfort is most specific and localized. Note the number and the name of the injury (on the illustration) that corresponds with this area. Based on the area of pain you've indicated, this is likely to be the correct diagnosis. However, remember that injuries often overlap! Therefore, I recommend that you don't leap to any conclusions. Follow through by doing *all* of the Bio-Point Exams. This will ensure the most accurate and informed assessment of your injury. To help guide you in determining your own injury, each exam includes typical comments from patients suffering from that particular injury.

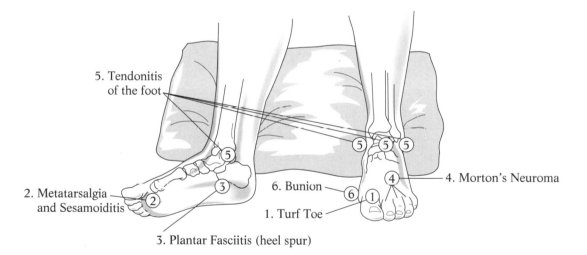

5. Tendonitis of the foot

4. Morton's Neuroma

2. Metatarsalgia and Sesamoiditis

6. Bunion

1. Turf Toe

3. Plantar Fasciitis (heel spur)

After each exam, the page number of the corresponding Med Unit is given. The Med Units are in Appendix A. Note: If no Med Unit is given, immediate, medical attention is advised—since the condition cannot be treated at home. By following the Med Unit instructions, you can begin treating your injury immediately, keeping close track of your progress as you go.

1. *Turf Toe*

COMMENTS: "My big toe hurts when I walk." "I've lost motion in my big toe."

EXAMS: Compare your toes. Does one have a hard ridge at the central joint? Press the ridge. Is there sharp, specific pain? Put yourself on tiptoes? Do you have sharp pain from the joint?

OTHER COMMENTS: This injury is commonly seen in football and tennis players.

THERAPY: see Med Unit, page 173.

2. *Metatarsalgia and Sesamoiditis*

COMMENTS: "The ball of my foot hurts." "I have trouble running."

EXAM/METATARSALGIA: Pinch the main joint of every toe—do any of them cause sharp pain?

EXAM/SESAMOIDITIS: Pinch the ball of the big toe between your fingers, bottom and top. Is there pain?

OTHER COMMENTS: These injuries are commonly caused by repetitive motion in sports such as running and ballet.

THERAPY: See Med Unit, page 173.

3. *Plantar Fasciitis (Heel Spur)*

COMMENTS: "My first few steps out of bed in the morning kill me. Then it gets better as the day goes on."

EXAM: Sit on a chair. Cross one leg to expose the heel. Press hard with a finger, probing the main area of the heel. Is there a searing pain in a specific area?

THERAPY: See Med Unit, page 174.

4. Morton's Neuroma

COMMENTS: "When I wear pointy shoes my feet hurt like crazy." "I get numbness and shocks in between two toes."

EXAM: Pinch the web space between the second and third, or third and fourth toes (occasionally this can affect the other toes as well). Does this create numbness and a radiating shock?

THERAPY: See Med Unit, page 174.

5. Tendonitits of the Foot

COMMENTS: "I've got a specific new pain in my foot." "I've recently changed my routine or training and now I have pain." "I've changed my running shoes (or street shoes) and have a new pain."

EXAM: Characteristically, tendonitis settles in one of three or four areas. Using the illustration (on page 113), press the foot at the indicated corresponding numbers. You can determine the location and severity of your condition by the amount of pain you experience.

THERAPY: see Med Unit, page 174.

6. Bunion

COMMENTS: "There is a lump on my big toe." "The joint of my big toe is red." "When I wear tight shoes, my big toe hurts."

EXAM: Inspect your naked foot. Is there a large bump on the inner part of the big toe? Flex the toe, and press down hard in the ridge of the foot. Is this painful?

THERAPY: See Med Unit, pages 174–175.

7. Stress Fracture of the Foot

COMMENTS: "The pain in my foot is not getting better." "I can't remember injuring myself."

THERAPY: A stress fracture of the foot is a lingering, unremitting, very severe pain which usually comes after a sudden excessive increase in exercise. If these are your symptoms, see a doctor.

9

Ankle

Two inches above the foot lies another "hot zone" for athletic injury: the ankle. Experts estimate a staggering 23,000 Americans sprain their ankles daily! I sometimes feel like I should have an annex in the Ankle Sprain Hall of Fame all to myself: I've been in six ankle casts; I've torn the ligaments in my left ankle four times; my right twice; I play permanently with braces in certain activities because I've got *laxity* in the ankle joint, meaning the ligaments are permanently stretched.

And I am, as I say, in good company, because ankle sprains are currently the most common of all acute sports injuries. The ankle brokers the stress between the ground-level push of the foot and the rest of the body, and though it is a sturdy customer, outfitted for its role, it still gets easily strained, and in worst-case scenarios, broken.

But it's not only acute injuries that bedevil this joint. With the recent boom in physical fitness, overuse injuries are becoming increasingly common, too.

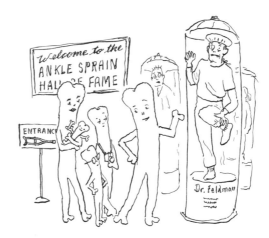

"Kids, this is the man with the most ankle sprains in the history of the world."

ANATOMY

A relatively primitive joint, the ankle has two main movements, levering the foot toward the shin (called, in med-speak dorsiflexion) and pointing the foot down and away in the opposite direction (called plantar flexion). To perform these motions the ankle draws on two major sets of ligaments and three major bones. The two main bones of the leg, the tibia and fibula, morph together at their bottom-most end to form the top half of the ankle joint. The ends of these bones form the characteristic ankle "knobs" we know and love (and bruise). These two knobs are held together by the *tibiofibular ligaments* (Figs 9.1 and 9.2).

The bottom half of the ankle joint is composed of the ankle bone itself, known as the *astragalgus*. This little fellow is unusual because, though a bona fide bone, it is without the usual muscles or tendon attachment. The astralgalgus exists to stabilize and firm the joint. It is enwrapped in ligaments. In fact, as befits a joint that is so directly on the firing line of athletic motion, the ankle is literally surrounded on all sides with tough ligamentous tissue—tissue calibrated to provide stability, but also loose enough to permit mobility.

It is that tissue, predictably enough, that is most often injured in sports.

INJURIES

Sprain

The ankle sprain sits atop the injury heap in sports, the hands-down winner for frequency of damage.

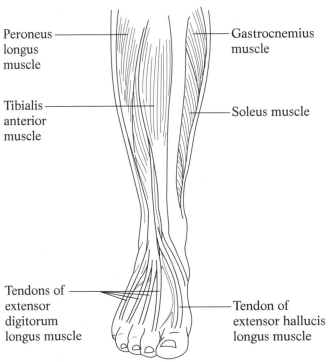

Peroneus longus muscle

Gastrocnemius muscle

Tibialis anterior muscle

Soleus muscle

Tendons of extensor digitorum longus muscle

Tendon of extensor hallucis longus muscle

Fig. 9.1 Front view of the ankle.

Ankle injuries run the gamut from stretch and tear, to complete rupture of the ligaments that keep the ankle bones in place, and keep you, correspondingly, up on your toes. Almost everyone, even if not an athlete, has "rolled" an ankle, with subsequent pain and swelling. Typically, uneven pavement, a divot in the grass of the playing field, a pothole in the road of the marathon, can cause these kinds of twists. But they are also common

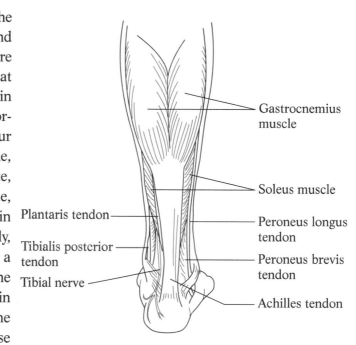

Fig. 9.2 Back view of the ankle.

among basketball players, who are jostling, often in midair, for possession of the ball. The main risk for an ankle sprain is that, if left untreated, it can lead to a chronically unstable condition, which can require major therapy and even surgery to cure.

When the ankle is tipped violently inward, it is called an *inversion sprain*. The first ligament to take the shock at such times is called the *anterior talofibular ligament*. When it gives up the ghost, the second ligament to take up the cause is the *calcaneal fibular ligament*, which runs from the outer ankle knob down to the heel bone. Obviously, a two-ligament sprain is more serious than a single-ligament version.

I've torn my ankle ligaments repeatedly. The first time I was in medical school, playing basketball with a now-famous orthopedic surgeon. He zigged, I zagged, I rolled my ankle over, and there was that fraction of a second in which I realized I'd been screwed. That "pop!" instantly lodged itself among my most painful memories. It was followed by the inevitable swelling of my ankle into something resembling a tangelo, accompanied by unbelievable pain.

Ankle Tendonitis

Overuse injuries to the ankle generally belong to the larger family of *tendonitis*, in some fashion. Two of the major culprits are the *outer* or *lateral*, ligaments, which terminate at the ankle, and—slightly less common—the *inner* or *medical* structures. Given the fancy name of **posterior tibial tendonitis**, this injury is commonly the result of overtraining and/or physical abnormalities to the foot such as pronation (see Chapter 7, pages 98–99), flat feet, or overly hard running surfaces.

Achilles Tendonitis

The Achilles tendon is the largest tendon in the body. Running down the back of the leg, about a foot and a half long, it terminates in the rear of the ankle. It is about the width of coaxial cable, and like a coaxial cable, is made up of multiple fibers, which is one of the reasons for its fantastic strength: it has been shown in tests to be able to withstand a torsion of 1,000 pounds. But despite its strength, Achilles tendonitis is a relatively common ankle-related difficulty, particularly among athletes who participate in running sports. And its likelihood increases sharply with age. (For those with a taste for history, an aside: the Achilles tendon is named after the mythical Greek warrior Achilles, who as a baby was dipped in a stream that rendered him invulnerable. Unfortunately for poor Achilles, it was the heel that he was held by as he was dipped, which made no contact with the stream, and was later pierced by an arrow, resulting in his death.)

Achilles tendonitis is a kind of "tennis elbow" of the lower leg. The tendon itself, due partly to its bulky size, is not particularly flexible, and sudden bursts of speed while running or the long-term wear and tear of years of jogging can cause microtrauma to the tendon that causes it to grow inflamed.

Achilles Tendon Tear

Occasionally the Achilles tendon is ruptured, producing one of the most devastating injuries in sports.

Typically, people who suffer an Achilles tendon tear say the same thing: I felt like I got shot in my heel. Often, in fact, you can hear a sound like a gunshot. I've seen it happen several times during ballet performances: the trademark loud crack! followed by the sickening slump to the floor of the afflicted dancer. But it can happen among even weekend athletes. I was playing basketball with friends once, and a pal was driving downcourt when he twisted his ankle and snapped his tendon. Suddenly we were all running for cover, certain that a basketball-hating sniper was on the loose.

A warning: continued Achilles tendon soreness is something to be looked at carefully since constant inflammation can change the microanatomy of the tendon, building up scar tissue, rendering the tendon less flexible, and predisposing it to rupture. The treatment is to cease the activity that causes the inflammation if possible; to stretch and do specific strengthening exercises; to ice the heel and tendon after you play; and to play with a heel lift in the shoe, which pulls the foot into a position of less stress. A cortisone injection is never indicated for Achilles problems, because it can, in fact, weaken the tendon. Most Achilles ruptures require surgery.

Healing Time with Ankle Strains

A lot of people come to my office two, three, four weeks after a strain, thinking that things will get better. Ankle strains take anywhere from six weeks to six months to recover from. It's a long convalescence. People are not educated about this, and assume a strain is something minor that goes away. It does, but only over time, and with proper treatment.

The good news is that few ankle strains require surgery, even when there's been a complete tear in the ligaments. In Europe, especially Sweden, the philosophy is to do surgery on nearly all ankle tears, whereas over here, we immobilize it so that the two broken ends kiss, and the ligament regrows.

Isn't that sweet?

The BIO-POINT Exam
A n k l e

PART ONE

Question 1
Is there any deformity in the afflicted area? Look in the mirror and if possible compare the affected and the unaffected side. Is there a lack of symmetry?
If "yes," see a doctor immediately.
If "no," read on.

Question 2
Is there a severe limitation in your range of motion? Are you incapable of performing basic household tasks with the afflicted extremity?
If "yes," see a doctor immediately.
If "no," read on.

Question 3
Is there any sign of extensive or excessive swelling?
If "yes," see a doctor immediately.
If "no," read on.

Question 4
Are you afflicted with severe weakness in the injured body part? Do you have difficulty for example, climbing stairs?
If "yes," see a doctor immediately.
If "no," read on.

Question 5
Was a loud "pop" heard at the time of the injury?
If "yes," see a doctor immediately.
If "no," read on.

PART TWO

Whew! You're still with me! That's very good news because it means your injury may fall within the guidelines of what is treatable at home. What I'm going to do now is to zero in on your problem and attempt to make a more accurate diagnosis. Look at the accompanying illustration and touch the area where your pain or discomfort is most specific and localized. Note the number and the name of the injury (on the illustration) that corresponds with this area. Based on the area of pain you've indicated, this is likely to be the correct diagnosis. However, remember that injuries often overlap! Therefore, I recommend that you don't leap to any conclusions. Follow through by doing *all* of the Bio-Point Exams. This will ensure the most accurate and informed assessment of your injury. To help guide you in determining your own injury, each exam includes typical comments from patients suffering from that particular injury.

After each exam, the page number of the corresponding Med Unit is given. The Med Units are in Appendix A. Note: if no Med Unit is given, immediate Medical attention is advised—since the condition cannot be treated at home. By following the Med Unit instructions, you can begin treating your injury immediately, keeping close track of your progress as you go.

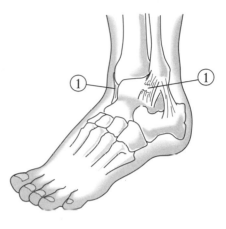

1. Sprains of the ankle

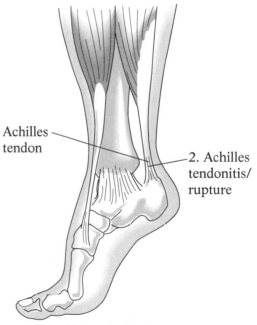

Achilles tendon

2. Achilles tendonitis/ rupture

Inside (medial) view

1. Sprains of the Ankle

COMMENTS: "I came down hard on my ankle and there was a pop." "I rolled my ankle and there was immediate swelling."

EXAM: Is there a large, swollen, black-and-blue mass around the ankle? This should be seen by a doctor immediately. If not, proceed to "therapy."

OTHER COMMENTS: This injury has been suffered by every basketball player on earth, and most volleyball players as well.

THERAPY: See Med Unit, page 175

2. Achilles Tendonitis/Rupture

COMMENTS/TENDONITIS: "The back of my ankle hurts when I run."

COMMENTS/RUPTURE: "It felt like I got shot in the heel."

EXAM: If there is a large purple gap at the back or your heel, see a doctor immediately. You have ruptured your Achilles tendon. Otherwise stand on the end of a stair and gradually lower your weight off the ball of your foot as you let your heel drop back. Do you feel acute pain or a dull ache throughout the Achilles tendon?

THERAPY: see Med Unit, page 175.

3. Osteochondritis Dissecans (Bone Chip)

COMMENTS: "My ankle sprain is not getting any better." "It's been six months and I still can't run."

EXAM: Sit in a chair. Raise your leg off the ground slightly and slowly flex your ankle forward, back, side to side. Is there a catching sensation? Ask yourself if there has been sustained swelling or the feeling of instability in the ankle—several month's worth.

THERAPY: See a doctor.

Part Three

Life Outside the Examining Room

10

Braces, Orthotics, and Footwear

To the uninitiated, the word orthotic sounds vaguely medical and threatening, a condition that might be the result of something traumatic: "I'm sorry ma'am, but your husband tripped and fell, and has become irreversibly orthotic." In fact, as most of you know quite well, an orthotic is either an off-the-shelf or custom-made device that is inserted in the shoe or sneaker and used to correct malalignment syndromes of various types. Properly employed, an orthotic will improve balance and athletic performance. The only problem with orthotics, as in so many things involving sports these days, is that orthotics have become big business, and with that boom has come the inevitable overuse and overprescription of the little wedges.

The fact is, not everybody with flat feet needs an orthotic. (See the boxed section on flat feet). Not everyone with pronation or rotation of the foot needs an orthotic. Orthotics will not correct male-pattern baldness or lack of stamina. What they can do is help center and align the body, and cut short some of the injury syndromes that begin at the feet and then often travel upward from there, spreading out in the familiar injury "cascade."

The point is that feet, in addition to levering the body forward, are the body's main shock absorbers. Whenever the action of those shocks is compromised up the leg, you get things like the dreaded *chondromalacia*, or knee soreness, and a variety of other unhappy difficulties. By being inserted correctly in the shoe, orthotics can help absorb that shock and keep you injury-free.

The Skinny on Flat Feet

Not everybody with flat feet needs orthotics, but flat feet is one of the conditions for which orthotics are most commonly prescribed. We've come a long way since the 1950s when flat feet were considered sufficient to keep someone out of the army. The generals believed that men with flat feet were incapable of long marches. And although flat feet, known medically as *pez plano valgus*, are often more vulnerable to fatigue, there are also cases of them being extremely athletic and durable. In general, flat feet are those in which the ligamentous structures are quite lax or loose. These feet have a tendency to form bunions at that apex of the foot, the big toe, where the stress of locomotion is concentrated. A *bunion* is the result of long-term steady-state irritation, which eventually causes an actual morphological change in the structure of the foot, with bone growth taking place at the joint, and that characteristic protrusive knob. The flat foot also often exhibits signs of pronation, in which the foot seems to fall inward, as the outer part of the foot rolls over slightly. In such instances, the stress of this malalignment travels up the leg to the next weakest link—the knee. Properly fitted and inserted, an orthotic can mimic the missing arch, and thereby "train" the foot into the correct position.

High arches tend to belong to inflexible feet, and produce a jarring shock of their own. Such feet often lead to shin splints (see Chapter 7, page 99). They are also good candidates for orthotics.

A big caveat emptor, or buyer beware here: most people with malalignment syndromes are asymptomatic anyway, and orthotics, improperly used, can sometimes create as many problems as they solve. Body types are endlessly individualistic, as are their problems. Buying an off-the-rack orthotic is like buying a pair of prescription glasses at a Home Depot. Better to bite the bullet, spend the time and the money, and go to a specialist in such things. You'll be glad you did.

BRACES

Is it me, or have braces become a fashion accessory just below navel rings in popularity? Time was, the brace was confined only to professional athletes, but nowadays these little neoprene (synthetic rubber) sleeves are everywhere you look.

A brace is an external mode of treatment designed to compensate for an internal weakness or malalignment. Obviously, a brace will not change the anatomy of a joint, but will "mind" it a bit, giving it crucial support. Ankle and knee braces are two of the most common, though there are also splints for wrists, elbows, shoulders, and ankles. An ankle brace, for example, is used to compensate for ligaments that, after many strains and or tears, have stretched. These ligaments will not, in and of themselves, return to normal. So a brace is applied, and surgery, hopefully, is avoided.

Ankle Braces

I know from ankle braces. Oh, boy, do I know. I'm the king of ankle sprains, and have worn more plaster on that little ball and socket than there is smoke in Gary, Indiana.

All of these sprains, by the way, are from basketball. My own opinion is that the technology of footwear hasn't yet caught up with the speed and violent movement inherent in the sport of basketball. Rarely, for example, does anyone survive a basketball career without sometimes severe

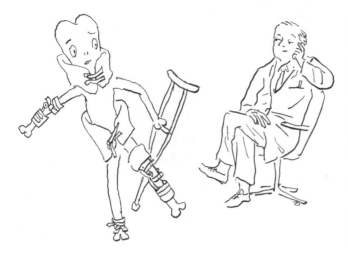

"Doc, I thought it was only an ingrown toenail!"

ankle sprains. The explosive start and stop of the game and the fact that you have to land from high jumps in a crowd of people, means that you twist and roll and give those ankles quite a beating along the way.

I play regularly in a league. All of us fellows are now in our midthirties and early forties and are essentially held together with glue and string. I noticed that when I started wearing an ankle brace, it quickly caught on. Soon, nearly all the other guys in the league were wearing them too. Needless to say, lost-player days were reduced immeasurably. The moral of the story: for certain kinds of ankle instability, braces work like a charm.

Essentially speaking, the ankle brace is used to recreate lost anatomy—cartilage, tissue, and mobility lost to wear and tear, age and arthritis. Some are just soft figure-eight braces, some are more rigid. Ankle braces are very individualistic, and above all should fit comfortably while serving their correct purpose. If you think you'd like to give one a try, I'd say go for it. However, before you pull one off the rack in your local sports shop, consult a physician first so you know you're getting a proper fit and a proper brace.

Knee Braces

Knee braces are much more complex and commonly prescribed than ankle braces. I'm sure everyone has seen them, ranging from a simple black neoprene sleeve, to the larger more complex constructions, that sometimes, with their rails and fabrics, look like something out of *Robocop*. All of them give extra support and warmth to the crucial joint of the knee. Some are used prophylactically, to ward off injury, and some are used post-injury, before or after surgery—most commonly for ACL tears. In my own research on this subject, I've found that the braces themselves—at least those trying to compensate for ACL tears—simply do not work. In general, if you're experiencing the knee instability and pain that comes with such a tear, you will instinctively stay away from a vulnerable situation (like a rough pickup basketball game). No brace will make you feel secure enough to risk it. However, knee braces can work more than adequately for other types of injuries. They are very specific in their function, and it is critical that you are prescribed the right one. Here are some various ones along with their uses.

> **The basic black sleeve.** As American as "the little black dress," this neoprene sleeve can add basic support and often helps with tendonitis.
>
> **The black sleeve with a hole in the center.** This is the *patella-bearing brace,* used for people *with chondromalacia* or *patella-femoral syndrome.*
>
> **Knee band or donut.** This foam-elastic brace encircles the patella tendon or kneecap and is specifically designed for patellar tendonitis.
>
> **Hinged braces.** This is used for damage to the medial or lateral ligaments of the knee.
>
> **Derotation braces.** This is the Robocop of braces, rigged out with all sorts of bells and whistles, which is used for ACL injuries.

There is a new and even larger brace just coming onto the market, by the way, which is designed specifically for arthritis of the knee and is showing promising results.

Other braces

> **Elbow brace.** This is an air pad or foam donut designed to take the stress off the tendon for "tennis" or "golfers" elbow.
>
> **Carpal tunnel brace.** This is a padded metal brace that puts the wrist in a position to alleviate the inflamed nerves.

Lumbar corset. This is a weight-lifting belt, which is designed to eliminate the pressure on the lumbar spine during sporting activities.

Cervical traction. This is used for neck strains and sprains.

FOOTWEAR

I could write an entire book on footwear. And yet everything I've learned
from a lifetime in competitive sports could be boiled down to one phrase:
stick with what works. This is harder to do than it appears. We're bombarded every day with glitzy ad campaigns for sneakers, each of them
promising a revolution in footwear and increased levels of athletic performance. Don't buy into it without
doing some careful research.

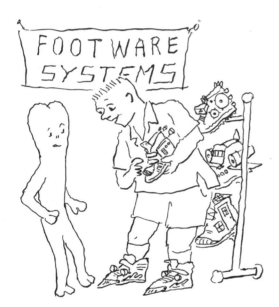

"This sneaker comes with a CD-ROM,
an instruction guide, and a zip code."

A case in point is what happened to me last year. I'd been running in a certain type of sneaker
pain-free for eight years. Swayed
by elaborate consumer ads, which
showed my favorite sporting figures soaring like grasshoppers and
pivoting like NBA versions of Fred
Astaire, I bit the bullet and bought
a different type of sneaker, more
expensive and boasting enough bells
and whistles to power Disneyworld.
Within two weeks I had pains in
places I never knew existed. Finally, after using my college degree
to narrow down the changes in my
routine, I targeted my sneakers. I
changed back to my basic unglamorous former sneakers and almost immediately my pains were gone. My original point bears repeating: *Go
with what got ya there.* The sneaker industry is big business and has a
vested interest in getting you to change what you wear. Don't believe the
hype. If what you have works for you, stick with it come hell or high water, the high cut, the low cut, the gel, the air, and the pump, too. The same

goes for basketball sneakers and golfing shoes. Be leery of changes made for the sake of fashion.

Some Footwear Points to Keep in Mind

• Never use a sneaker actively for more than six months and expect it to still cushion you when you jump or run. Sneakers lose their cushioning rapidly, and lose their stability as well. Certain sneakers lose their cushioning faster than others. Inform yourself before you buy.

• In general, sneakers with black rubber bottoms last longer than those with white bottoms.

• When a sneaker gets wet, and then sits, the materials of that sneaker can change their texture and consistency. If your sneaker does get wet, remove the insole, and then stuff it with shape-retaining old rags or newspaper until it dries. Never ever employ a clothes drier, as you're sneakers will lose their elasticity and will shrink drastically.

• If you're buying a sneaker for running, then know in advance what type of material you'll be running on. Cinder tracks are best; asphalt or blacktop are second best; concrete is the least absorbtive and therefore the least desirable. Choose the shoe accordingly.

• Buy in a runner's store whenever possible; the sales people are always more informed.

• If you're a pronator, request a shoe with more *motion control.*

• If you're heavy, ask for a shoe with as much absorbtive potential as possible. Every step you take while running hits the ground with anywhere from four to eight times your body weight.

11

Women and Sports

I'm now going to step forward, clear my throat, and make an earth-shattering announcement: women are different from men. I know, I know, it's a self-evident truism, something like saying, "the earth is round," or "the sky is blue." But in these days of identity politics, there is so much tension in pointing out the differences between things that most people shrink from saying the obvious. So I'll say it again. Women are different from men: biologically, neurologically, skeletally, and even chemically. Their pelvises are larger. They menstruate. Their bones are lighter and the fibers of their muscles are more delicate. Unfortunately, they often come to sports later in life so their muscle balance can sometimes be off, which predisposes them to certain injuries.

Interestingly, when it comes to sports involving the lower extremities, women can come

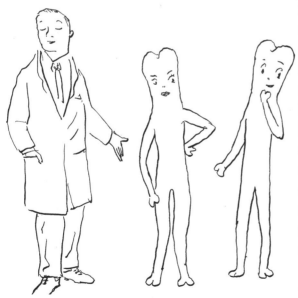

"My homeroom teacher was right: there is a difference between girls and boys."

pretty close to men in performance, as the current history of the marathon demonstrates quite conclusively. I have played most sports with women, and have found that they approach men's level of performance in soccer, bike riding, running, and skiing—to take four.

The last misperception that needs correcting is that men are a hundred times more involved in sports than women. There are, statistically, many more men involved in sports than women, but the last ten years have witnessed radically increased levels of women's participation in nearly every sport you can name—with the exception perhaps, of rock-em sock-em contact sports like ice hockey and football. The WNBA is just a flag blowing in the wind from the future: women's sports are now big business and here to stay.

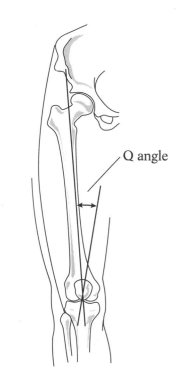

Fig. 11.1 Measuring the Q angle.

INJURIES

Women athletes run certain specific risks and have a characteristic tendency toward certain ailments. I'll sketch them in briefly here.

Runner's Knee

The wider pelvis of a woman causes the knees to be more knocked (creating what is known as the Q angle), which can cause the feet to splay out, and the kneecaps to slide out of their grooves (Fig 11.1). Research also tends to indicate that the groove in which the kneecap sits is shallower in women than in men: you put that all together and it spells patella problems—patella-femoral syndrome.

Tennis Elbow

I have heard, though I haven't seen it much personally, that women develop this more often than men, as a result of weaker forearm development. See Chapter 4, pages 52–54 for more details on this epidemic difficulty.

Stress Fractures

These are the bane of many serious female athletes, and for a specific reason. Women, particularly those who practice endurance sports like the marathon, tend to develop menstrual irregularities. If they are already thin, they often suffer from *dysmenorrhea*, which is an erratic menstrual cycle. These metabolic stresses are worsened by the fact that according to studies, anywhere from 15 to 62 percent of female athletes have eating disorders.

The result—a menstrual cycle gone haywire—has far-reaching metabolic consequences. With the interruption of the menstrual cycle, hormone production drops. And because hormones specifically condition bone growth (estrogen is crucial in allowing calcium to be absorbed from the intestines), those bones grow brittle and weak. An astonishing 50 percent of competitive female runners with irregular periods suffer stress fractures.

Women who experience irregular periods while training should first of all be honest with themselves about eating disorders. Body fat is crucial to producing periods, and it is possible that an eating disorder or an undiagnosed tendency to anorectic behavior is exacerbating the condition. They should quiz themselves specifically about their protein intake, as studies suggest a correlation between protein intake and *amenorrhea* or lack of periods. Also to be determined: the percentage of total calories from fat. This should hover around 20 percent. As a general rule of thumb, calcium supplements should be taken, and if the athlete eats a very high fiber diet, it should be remembered that high fiber can sometimes act to flush calcium from the system.

A perfect example of the ways in which eating disorder can exact a hidden toll on a woman athlete's body is the case of someone I'll call

Sarah. Sarah was a glamorous character who I knew from my gym. She was a serious recreational runner, and she began to suffer an intractable hip pain. She dragged herself from doctor to doctor, each of whom x-rayed the hip and then told her not to worry about it. She was meanwhile running excessively, eating badly, vomiting often. She had a stress fracture but no one ever diagnosed it—remember, these are tricky to spot on a regular X-ray. By the time it was detected, it was too late. She required an entire hip replacement—and at the ripe old age of thirty-two!

The pelvis, hip, thigh, shin, and back of female athletes are the places that are most likely to suffer from stress fractures. Female gymnasts are particularly prone to stress fractures of the lumbar spine. In the worst cases, one vertabrae slides over another, the nerves are impinged upon, and the back must be fused.

The hormonally related weakening of bones and subsequent difficulties is THE single most troubling diagnosis we're seeing on the new wave of female athletes. The upside? Regular exercise has been proven to minimize the scalding discomforts of PMS and periods generally. The endorphins flooding the body cut down on the aches and cramps, and the tonic aerobic effects tend to relax the mind.

Urinary-Tract Problems

For a variety of reasons, women have a generally higher chance of getting urinary-tract infections than men. For female athletes, this is yet another reason why hydration is so important: the constant washing out of the bladder and urethra tends to improve resistance to infection. On the other hand, women athletes experience more problems with incontinence than men. Often, pregnancy leaves the pelvic muscles stretched, with the result that there is a bit less bladder control than previously. Pelvic-contraction exercises (known as kegels) will generally bring this under control.

Nutritional Note: women athletes need a higher concentration of iron in their blood than men do. The combination of exercise and menstruation means that iron supplements are usually required.

Breasts

The sports bra has been a revolution in the war against breast discomfort during jogging and other sports. Nipple irritation is still sometimes a problem, but can be minimized by taping or Band-Aiding the nipple, to reduce chafing. When trying on a bra, try to run in place or do jumping jacks for a minute or so, to properly evaluate the support and comfort of the bra.

Pregnancy

I wouldn't recommend a woman in her third trimester undertake the triple jump event, but moderate exercise is safe until a relatively advanced stage of pregnancy. Women who are athletically inclined, and practice prudent, regular exercise during their pregnancy, generally recover their former physiques more quickly than sedentary women. There are some who say that labor time is reduced and made easier, though no studies demonstrate this conclusively.

In 1985, the American College of Obstetricians and Gynecologists (ACOG) released guidelines on exercise during pregnancy and the post-partum period. Most of these are reasonably obvious, and involve moderate amounts of exercise, the avoidance of deep flexion or extension of joints, careful hydration, and the monitoring of proper caloric intake

12

Medical Testing Today: What You Can Expect

Medical science in America has come a long way in a short time. A scant two hundred years ago, doctors still believed that convulsing the patient through a variety of purges and bloodlettings was the fastest road to health. The father of our country, George Washington was drained of a quart and a half of Presidential blood on the day of his death—a treatment that certainly hastened his demise. Thank god those days are behind us! But the fundamental precepts of medicine are the same now as then: diagnosis is made after all the information has been gathered and sifted. This information is collected with elbow grease, observation, deductive instinct, and often a dose of intuition thrown in for good measure. For doctors, the equation is simple: knowledge is power. Our role, on the diagnostic side of things, is the humble one of gathering information, the better to aim the magic bullet of our cure.

And yet there are obviously many times when direct observation is not enough, when the best eyes and hands in the world can't tell you what you need to know. This is when that little thing called technology rides to the rescue. The doctor of today has access to a fantastic array of tests to "see" inside the body. To the uninitiated, these are an intimidating stew of letters: MRI, CAT scan, EKG, and so forth. And, it has to be admitted that they are sometimes overused, for reasons of laziness on the part of doctors. Often, too, they are demanded by patients who have seen or read about them, who want the bells and whistles, or who, in a bizarre form of celebrity worship, have learned that their favorite athlete had one, and feel that being bombarded with high-performance electrons will allow them to feel "close" to their chosen superstar. Occasionally they are used as decision makers by insurance companies to allow a doctor to treat a patient in a certain way. My own opinion, as someone who relies on them regularly, is that, on balance, high-technology diagnostics are probably a bit overused. Not everybody needs to have these kinds of tests; there is no substitutes for good old-fashioned elbow grease and deductive instinct. Nonetheless, in the interests of clarity, I'll give you a brief guide to some of the more advanced observational technologies the next orthopedic surgeon might use on you.

X RAY

This is the classic—a kind of American heirloom technology, the Norman Rockwell modality of diagnostic medicine. An X ray is a radiologic test that, under proper circumstances, emits a level of radiation to your body that is the equivalent of spending an hour in the sun. It basically shows the bone and only the bone, allowing a doctor to determined if it's fractured, arthritic, or dislocated. The bone and the joint are seen quite clearly, but nothing else is. When you want to investigate the health of soft tissue like tendons, ligaments, nerves, and vessels, you have to go elsewhere, because the X ray is no use.

MRI

The MRI actually stands for *magnetic resonance imaging*, but it might as well stand for Most Requested Investigation. The MRI is a wonderful tool, which allows one to peer into the body noninvasively, and without subjecting the body to any negativity. But it has rapidly become the Elvis of high-tech diagnostics, a cult tool that is routinely requested by people who think it will solve their problems or give them new leases on life. The MRI is a serious piece of breakthrough technology, which can do certain things better than they've ever been done before. But it is not a cure-all, nor is it a replacement for careful observation and deduction on the part of doctors.

The MRI doesn't use radiation in the conventional sense. Rather, it combines the use of a large magnet and radio waves. The hydrogen atoms in the patient's body react to the magnetic field, and a computer analyzes the results and makes pictures of the inside of the body. The images are of astonishing clarity.

An MRI cuts a 360-degree picture, "slicing" the injury site in a variety of directions and allowing unparalled access to the inside of the body. Not only the bones seen in X rays, but all soft-tissue details—all swellings, tumors, rips of tendons, ligagments, and vessels—are seen in vivid clarity. There are two reasons why people don't like MRIs. They think it causes them pain and they incur radiation. Neither of these are true. However, claustrophobia is an issue, among those who suffer from the fear of being enclosed in confined spaces, because you have to be inserted in a large tube-shaped housing for about a half-hour and remain entirely motionless. But newer models are slightly less forbidding.

CAT SCAN

This stands for *computerized axial tomography*, which though it sounds like a missile-guidance system, in fact describes the technology the CAT scan uses to take pictures of the body's interior. CAT scans are similar to the MRI, but instead of using a magnet, it uses a radiation technique. Though the CAT scan has been superseded by the MRI, it's still good for some things: a little better at seeing bone, a little poorer at seeing soft tissue.

THE EMG

Known as *electrical myelography* in the parlance, this procedure involves taking an electrical wire and using it to test nerves, in the same way a circuit tester is used to determine why your CD player is on the fritz. It is employed only for determining the extent and location of nerve damage. I often liken the problem with nerves to a phone line: if you're calling and there's ice on the line, the connection will be poor or nonexistent. The EMG allows us to find that "ice," a disturbance that often doesn't show on an MRI. The plus side of things is that the EMG is very accurate. The downside is they are slightly invasive, employing what's called a filament needle somewhat like an acupuncture needle, to prick the skin.

These are the major tests, the ones you are most likely to encounter. As important as they are, they are less important than the experience, intellect, and intuition of your doctor.

13

New Treatments in Sports Medicine

My dream for the future of medicine is that it continues to evolve as quickly a sit has over the last twenty years. Many treatments are now available that were unthinkable two decades ago. Ideally, the doctor one day will be the medical equivalent of a very good cat burglar: he slips in, slips out, and leaves the house (or patient) undamaged.

And yet, of course, that's not something we'll likely see—at least not in my lifetime. No, doctors invariably change things in the process of curing people. And we surgeons alter the equation of the body with every cut we make. If I reconstruct the ligament of a knee, I have to take another piece of tissue to compensate for that—which creates a subtle but irreversible change in the body. When I rebuild a shoulder, I cut and reconstruct and overlap—and change the anatomy in the process.

New treatments and trends in sports medicine are proliferating everywhere in professional athletics—from the *hyperbaric* (oxygen) *chambers* in which injured athletes lie to speed up healing to the little Breath-Rite nose-clips that many sports figures now wear to keep the nasal passages open and encourage oxygen intake; from biofeedback and visualization and guided imagery to nutritional counseling. In my own field of orthopedic surgery, medical innovations generally have two aims: to reduce the disruption of the surgery itself and speed up recovery times.

Which brings us to the arthroscope—a device that has revolutionized orthopedic surgery in our time. I'm a car nut, so I'll use an automo-

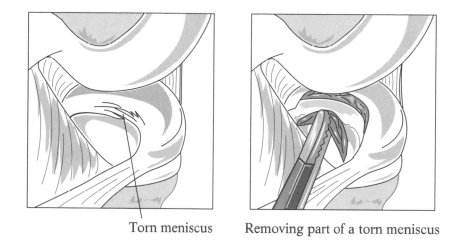

Torn meniscus   Removing part of a torn meniscus

Fig. 13.1 Arthroscopic surgical removal of a torn meniscus.

tive figure of speech here: to change a taillight, you don't need to tunnel through the front grill all the way to the back to make the repair. You enter the site of the damage as locally and discreetly as possible, do what you need to do, and disappear. Which is exactly why the arthroscope is such a wonderful invention.

When a person gets "scoped," he or she is benefiting from the perfect fusion of videotechnology and engineering prowess. The arthroscope is a steel wand that contains a tiny television camera and microfilament lighting in its nose, which is placed in the afflicted joint and broadcasts the inner workings of that joint with remarkable clarity on a color television monitor.

Live, from you're knee, it's Dr. Feldman!

Working with other wands containing small shavers, snippers, and gobblers, the doctor cleans cartilage, reconstructs ligaments, stops dislocations, does just about everything but take dictation, it seems (see Fig. 13.1) By entering the body through a pinhole aperture rather than an incision, the arthroscope imposes minimum trauma on the area. Discomfort is reduced, and healing time is slashed significantly. This same technology is currently used in other parts of the body, in spinal operations, and in gynecological surgery, to name two.

The only drawback of arthroscopic surgery is that the expertise to do these techniques takes a long time to develop. To my patients, I liken arthoscopic technique to the miniature crane in the toybox at the penny arcade: you can't just reach in and get the fuzzy bear by hand; no, you have to develop the dexterity and an extra tactile sense that is not god-given.

That said, the last ten years have seen a further refinement of the already minimally invasive techniques of the arthroscope. Originally used only for work on the *meniscus* of the knee—plucking out damaged tissue—it is now used for a wide variety of diagnostic and surgical procedures involving every joint of the body. Obviously, as stated, the goal is to leave no trace at all, to play God as it were, perfectly reconstructing a functioning system.

The magic silver wand of the arthroscope is waving us toward a medical future that looks exceedingly bright. We're currently close to realizing the science-fiction-flavored fantasy of cartilage regeneration: taking cells that are blank slates and putting these cells in specific juices, sauces, and broths while growing them into exactly what we want them to be—and then implanting them and thereby recreating structures exactly as they were before they were damaged. I'm involved with these projects, and I can assure you that there will one day be a time, in the not too distant future, where I'll be able to tell my patients, "I've cured your arthritis." Or, "don't worry, we'll grow you another ligament for your knee."

As wondrous as cartilage regeneration is, it is merely the tip of the research iceberg. Cloning may allow us to cure cancer, to restore spinal-cord injuries, to potentially reverse aging, in fact. Fatigue-free composite metal implants may allow joint replacements that are close to natural functioning—a long awaited dream of hip-replacement patients. Capsular shrinkage techniques will change things on a cellular nature and permit shrinkage and contraction of tissue, banishing those laxity problems that so often afflict joints. Lipotripsy, an ultrasonic sound-and-water treatment currently used to pulverize kidney stones, may soon come on board to treat those intractably difficult heel spurs.

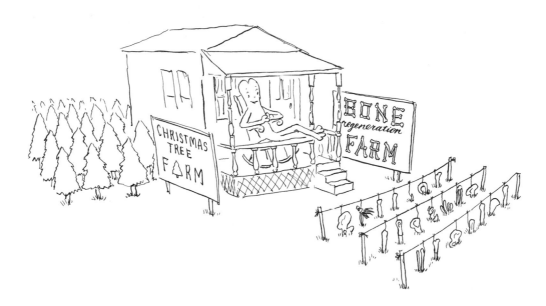

"They said it couldn't be done, but it will be, and soon."

14

Sports Medical Nutrition

Have you ever noticed how astonishing are the improvements in athletic performance over the last twenty or thirty years? The fastest men's marathon from 1960 wouldn't have even placed in the top three of our most recent *women's* marathon. The same "then" and "now" disparity is in every field of athletic endeavor: coaching and technical support for athletes grows increasingly sophisticated, and the performance blooms. But there are reasons aside from improved training methods and gear that people are constantly smashing athletic records. A key one is the recent increase in our understanding of the metabolic and chemical processes of the body, and with that, a deepened realization of the importance of nutrition. Up until a decade or so ago, the only nutritional advice for athletes was: Eat a lot! These days, specific diets rich in differing ratios of fats, proteins, carbohydrates, and sugars are now recommended for specific athletic events. Athletes in endurance sports, for example, generally do better with a high-carb low-protein diet, which is why you see marathoners bolting pasta before a race. Athletes in sports requiring brute strength tend to build those bulging muscles with a more protein-oriented input.

Then there's fat. Americans from that point of view, are not a pretty people. The combination of indolence and fast-food restaurants has rendered us the most upholstered race on the planet. Odd to realize, then, that fat is actually an important part of the body's nutritional system, and serves as the most concentrated source of energy we possess. In addition to its insulating and shock-absorbing properties, fat provides a transport system for certain vitamins through the body, and supplies essential fatty acids as well. Fat should be about 10–30 percent of your daily caloric intake.

I'm a vegetarian, myself, not for any high-flown political reason, but because I don't like the taste of meat. Also, I have to say that the sight of the many clogged arteries and fat-choked hearts I saw in anatomy class as a med student tended to spur me pretty seriously toward the greens. I was once consulting at a health spa when the nurse there showed me what they used to scare people off fatty diets: human fat, a grotesque yellow and pink five-pound plastic bag of it, marbled with serosanguineous ooze. I can guarantee that if you keep this baby on your kitchen table, your calorie intake will drop right off the charts! Personally, I sin with cheese, which I can't get enough of, and pasta, which is my private god. But I haven't had a piece of meat in twenty years. Though this causes me the occasional awkward moment at steakhouses and certain fancy restaurants, it's become a way of life. If you're considering a vegetarian lifestyle, here's something that might help nudge you in the right direction: massage experts say that the muscles of vegetarians, believe it or not, actually feel smoother and more supple than those of people who eat meat!

SUPPLEMENTS

Because we live in a trend-oriented society, and because our health is so important to us, we're bombarded on every side with advice, sales pitches, and commercials for diets and nutritional supplements. You can take saw palmetto oil for your prostate, dong kwai or ginseng for your flagging sex drive, vitamin A for your bad eyesight, shark cartilage for your immune system, and melatonin to help you sleep at night. A chaser of gingko biloba will help you remember all the checks you wrote at the vitamin store that week. Unfortunately, medical science offers no hard evidence that you can improve your athletic performance with these glamorous-sounding additives. Also, let's face it, these materials are big business, and you can easily go broke believing, and buying into, the assorted claims.

On the one hand, the placebo effect is real. If you believe something will help you, it often will. Once in my life I took a sleeping pill. As I drifted off on an instantaneous river of relaxation, I thought, "Wow, this is amazing! I've never felt so peaceful in my life!" The next morning I learned I'd taken an over-the-counter antacid. On the other hand, things like ginseng and certain Chinese herbal additives *will* give you increased energy. But so will a cup of coffee. Recent studies, in fact, indicate that coffee will definitely enhance athletic performance and allow you to cheat fatigue a little. (This corroborates perfectly with my memory of Italian skiing star Alberto Tomba, who in the timing shed just before starting his gold-medal run, knocked back an espresso with his gloves on and his pinkie finger sticking out. I thought it was just a charming affectation at the time: but no, there was good medicine behind that caffeine).

Obviously, most of us are not concerned with shaving hundredths of a second off our downhill runs; we want the nutritional input that will allow us to sleep better, play injury-free longer, keep our energy up. The debate over vitamin and mineral supplements is unending. Use your intuition. Remember, in a perfect state of nature, we wouldn't need any supplementary vitamins or minerals. But things like alcohol, coffee, stress, and cigarettes deplete the body of specific essential minerals and vitamins, and in such cases it may not be a bad idea to try to balance your biological checkbook and put them back into the account.

15

Alternative Medicine and Sports

When President Clinton, in his first term, appointed a commissioner of Alternative Medicine, it merely crystallized what a lot of people in the country had felt for a long time: that there were other valid approaches to health and well-being than the classic Western model. Times have changed, and even the most conventional Western doctors now have to admit that the naturopathic and Eastern ways have something to teach us. If you need proof of this, take the Chinese: Their medicine has been around for five thousand years, and their current population of about a billion would tend to argue they know what they're doing!

The world really *is* a global village. In Italy, American basketball stars are revered with an intensity that rivals the Pope's. Japanese is now spoken in the New York Yankee locker room, and in the Tokyo Dome, you can hear American guys in the dugout trying to say "Rosin bag" in their strange new language. Baby-boomer America has embraced alternative medicine enthusiastically, and I say: more power to 'em. That's right. It's nearly the year 2000 and it's really time to have an open mind.

Unfortunately, not *all* doctors feel this way. A substantial portion of the American medical establishment still believes that if a problem doesn't show up on an X ray or a throat culture it doesn't, fundamentally, exist. And yet these same doctors have to concede that the laws of healing are finally mysterious ones, conditioned by intangibles such as outlook, enthusiasm, and that vague but powerful thing, "the will to live." I've had patients who should have been on crutches for months after knee surgery come jogging happily by me on the street three weeks later. And others, of the exact same age and physical specifics, who take three times as long to heal.

American medicine leads the world in treating infection and in soft- and hard-tissue repair, but as I see it, Western doctors can still benefit from exposure to new ideas. They can learn to be open-minded and more attuned to the emotional context of illness. They can better understand the fundamental interactivity of all the different systems of the body. They can grow beyond being mere technicians. And they can use these alternative philosophies in their own work. Here are some quick hits on the most popular alternative-medicine regimens of the moment.

Alternative Treatments

Speaking generally, alternative treatments attempt to promote healing and recovery with as little organic disruption as possible. Some treatments currently in vogue are:

Yoga One of the very best things for people suffering from stiffness, muscle weakness, and often, emotional problems, too. I recommend it regularly for patients. It has evolved well past the hand-holding mystical phase of once upon a time. Look for hatha yoga, which is classical yoga, and in particular iyengar yoga, which is a very tough, deep, intelligent yoga. Those more athletically inclined may want to try ashtanga yoga, a moving, jumping yoga, which will have you sweating and panting hard. This is sometimes advertised as "power yoga."

Massage Massage is without peer in rejuvenating tired muscles and giving an overall tonic to the body. As those *Great American Backrub* stores testify, massage has caught on big time in America. I often send patients for massage. There are many varieties:

    Swedish-Style Massage. This is the classic massage. Make sure the massage therapist is a licensed practitioner. This is a good all-purpose massage, useful for soreness and body aches and general stress.

Medical Massage. This is a deep massage specifically targeted at frozen or knotted areas. This is not a general body massage, and is usually given only in conjunction with a medical treatment.

Reflexology. This is an intriguing and effective massage centered on the feet but working the internal organ systems through what are called trigger points: specific nerve endings on the feet. I've had this done, and the results are quite wonderful.

Rolfing. This is a very serious deep-muscle massage. It is based on the concept that muscles have memories and have frozen in response to trauma. Based on the discoveries of Ida Rolf, a Swiss doctor who invented the techniques to save her crippled son, it is sometimes incandescently painful, as the practitioners separate the muscle from its fascia, or outer fibrous sheath. But there are many who swear by it, and label its results "life changing."

Polarity balancing. This is a massage that tries to "reroute" the essential energy flow of the body. This gets into grey areas that seem nearly mystical to a hardheaded scientist, but again, there are many people who claim that polarity-balancing massage has given them new energy, and allowed them to overcome emotional problems.

Craniosacral. This is a massage that works on readjusting the plates of the skull, the areas where the skull meets the neck, and something called "the cerebrospinal pulse." For a fascinating discussion of this kind of massage, read the third chapter of Dr. Andrew Weil's book, *Spontaneous Healing.*

Acupressure/Shiatsu. This is a favorite of many patients. This massage employs the same 5,000-year-old map of energy meridians as acupuncture, and relies on specific pressure on nerve points to promote an overall invigoration and toning. This is less useful for specific muscle trauma.

Massage, as I say, is wonderful for the body. The only downside of it is that it's entirely passive, and the results only last a few days.

Some Other Alternative Treatments

Magnet Therapy. This is an oft-disputed healing regimen that supposedly works by stirring up the energy field and attracting blood and healing elements to the area. Magnets are now being used by the NFL in certain healing situations. On this subject, stay tuned, as it's about to open up wide.

Biofeedback. This is a self-induced hypnotic state, arrived at through a meditation-style technique. Biofeedback is very useful for lowering blood pressure, and is particularly recommended for migraine-sufferers.

Fasting. All the rage at certain health spas, fasting can give a body a break, and allow it some downtime, during which, so the fasting logic runs, it can clean itself out. Fasters report the first day and a half or so are intensely difficult, but after that, the hunger pains pass, and a kind of exhiliration arrives. Fasting should only be tried with great care and preferably under supervision, if for more than a day.

Aromatherapy. This is another standby at spas. In this treatment people either breathe medicinal herbs, or are daubed with solutions of them, and are then enfolded in hot wet blankets. Users report a feeling of great serenity afterward. Myself, I prefer beer.

Chiropractic. This is a booming field, but one without a lot of oversight. Point being: there are good ones and bad ones. Anyone in theory can hang up a shingle. Make sure yours comes both licensed and carefully recommended. Chiropractic suffers from the same fate as massage: because it is done to you, and you are not learning any new behaviors, your body will sooner or later revert to its old ways. That's why chiropractic, in conjunction with yoga, is an even better idea.

These are some of the main alternative treatments, but the truth is there are dozens more, some reputable, some not. The best thing to do before you undertake any of them is to inform yourself. Health-food stores bristle with books on these subjects, and, if you have a computer, the World Wide Web is full of sites with relevant information.

16

Alternative Sports and Their Common Injuries

When I was a boy I had a skateboard. It was a thin slip of wood with skinny wheels, and I floated gingerly on it up and down the gentle grades around my house. It was fun, it was faintly daring, and the worst that could happen was I'd skin a knee. Flash-forward thirty years to a dread-locked teen idol on a "pro-slick longboard" who is "floating a fat ollie" off the ramp before a screaming crowd. Under what rock have I been sleeping for these past three decades?

To the Gen X-ers who invented them, alternative sports were the quickest way out from under the stifling restrictions of traditional athletics with its uniforms and schedules and the endless fine print of its rules. "Day-Glo *this*!" shouted a legion of young MTV-watchers in the '80s, streaming out of the stadiums and playing fields and onto the roads and rockfaces and beaches of America en masse, and in the process, changing the face of sports in this country forever. The great thing about alternative sports is they get you out *there*, in nature, fast, and at the same time provide the oxygen jolt of some hairy extremes: bungee jumping, mountain biking, and snowboarding, to name three.

When you take the wide view (my favorite view as I grow older), it's easy to see that alternative sports are part of a larger recent trend toward athletic risk-taking in this country. I don't think it can be denied by anyone that athletic thrill-seeking, suddenly, is all the rage.

Take Extreme Sports. Have you heard of it? Extreme Sports is a species of organized mayhem that overlaps alternative sports on the lunatic fringe, and has been described as "any sport that requires three Hail Mary's before first attempting it, and consumes two-third's the body adrenaline in a single shot." Cliff diving, free climbing, sky surfing, wake boarding, near-vertical face skiing: there was always an element of danger in sport, of course, but nothing like there is today, where actively, dynamically taunting fate is part of the bargain. The Extreme Games, ESPN's televised Olympics of the death-defying, is showing huge growth among TV watchers eager for cheap thrills, and adventure-vacations where danger is part of the package are some of the hottest tickets in tourism today: off-road cycling, shark diving, sea kayaking, heli-skiing, to name a few. These are expensive vacations, obviously, undertaken most often by people considerably older than Generation X. A specific example: Outward Bound, the rugged wilderness training course, reported an explosive 66 percent rise from 1992 to 1996 in *executive participation*. Why these good people would want to leave their climate-controlled offices for the opportunity to wake up in the Arctic tundra being tongue-washed by a grizzly bear is beyond me, but so be it.

INJURIES

Though alternative sports promotes some entirely new sporting hardware, and uses entirely new techniques in certain cases, the body in question is the old familiar standby, and it fractures and strains and bruises accordingly. The following are some typical alternative sports and their typical injuries.

Mountain Biking

Once upon a time it was a bicycle built for two, with Burt Bacharach music in the background and a calm breeze in your face. Now its's gear-wrenching, mud-wrestling, knobby-tired madness, with the adrenaline pumping and riders yanking themselves up and down hills at high speed. The most serious injuries I see from mountain and off-road bicycling are obviously head injuries, which can be cut down drastically with the simple specific of a helmet. If you're out on a mountain-bike course without a helmet, you're already clinically insane, and can stop reading here. The

Rollerblading

The Rollerblade or in-line skate deserves an entry of its own because it's the essential symbol of the alternative revolution in sports, and did as much to usher in a change in our athletic habits as the Sony Walkman did our enjoyment of music. Currently the single fastest growing of all recreational sports, Rollerblading is no longer really "alternative" to anything, unless it's walking. Why has it become so popular? Because the Rollerblade is a good thing: relatively cheap, efficient, eco-friendly, and better at lifting confirmed couch spuds off their duffs and into the sunshine than any other piece of sporting equipment you can name. I should know. I've been jogging the same outdoor trails in Central Park for fifteen years, and on sunny days bladers now outnumber runners. Most of them, of course, know their business and are quite able to zig and zag fluently, but I worry about the ones who are obviously beginners—the ones I see so often, tottering and jerky, dressed in skintight spandex and trying to smile through their terror, windmilling their arms as if taxiing for takeoff and ending up, as often as not, flat on their backs. In-line skating is not a risk-free sport. After all, if for some reason your talent in basketball isn't the finest and your reflexes are off a tick, you miss a shot. But if your athletic talent on blades isn't up to par, especially in New York City, it can cost you a fortune in dental work!

rest of you should know that a specific group of mountain-biking injuries occur when the rider falls over the handlebars, landing on the shoulder to brace the impact, and thereby adding **shoulder separations** and **dislocations** to the mix. Depending on what piece of anatomy you brace your fall with, your wrists and elbows may also be effected.

As for me, I was happy with the daring look of my Stingray bicycle in gradeschool and kind of left things there. But my appetite has been whetted by the mountain-bike revolution. For those who do ride, here are some tips to avoid spilling yourself all over the trail.

First and most simply: **look ahead**, forward, and into the future, not down and at the present. At 15 miles an hour, you should be scanning the view about 50 to 75 feet ahead of you—anticipating, in a word. Looking ahead also has the advantage of straightening your stressed-out back, and giving it a break. Experts advise that the best way to go downhill fast while remaining in control is to **stand on the pedals and lean slightly back**, squeezing the seat between the thighs. Push the bike ahead of you slightly to get your weight back. When going uphill, **crouching while pulling the handlebars toward you** tends to lower your all-important center of gravity without causing the rear wheel to lose traction.

Sooner of later, whether you're a wild mountain biker or a docile two-wheeler, you're going to fall. Tips when falling:

Toss the Bike The majority of accidents occur when the unforgiving steel geometry of the bike tangles on the ground with your soft body parts. If you fall, get as far away from that angry piece of metal as possible! Let it move forward or leave it behind.

Assume a Tuck Once the bike has lost its way and it's clear you're launching airborne, experts advise to "think like a ball"—assume a tuck as best you can, bringing your arms and feet in toward your chest. This tends to minimize breaking those precious extremities.

Roll The best thing to do is make like a stone and turn end over end, preferably in the tuck position. Rolling—as opposed to sliding—tends to minimize friction and maximize things like your clothes and your skin.

Rollerblading

Rollerbladers tend to have specific injuries, which range form simple sprains to the unfunny fact of death. Typical injuries include **wrist fractures, knee sprains, shoulder dislocations** and **fractures,** and **head**

trauma. Apart from knowing what you're doing, gauging the terrain and traffic patterns to your ability, never "skitching" as it's called (hitching a ride on a moving vehicle), and making sure your equipment and brain is in working order, the best thing you can do to cut down on injuries is wear protective gear.

Protective Gear

A **helmet** is a good start, of course, but there's more to it than that. No less august a governing body than the *International In-Line Skating Association* recommends the use of serious protective measures when blading: a helmet, sure, but **wrist guards**, and **knee** and **elbow pads** to boot. They recommend these measures because they work. For bladers, skaters, and skateboarders, the delicate wrist is a particular weakpoint. Wrist guards have been proven to be highly effective not merely against hyperextension of the wrist, but against laceration, too. Wrist guards reduce the odds of sustaining a wrist injury sixfold, according to a recent study. Knee and elbow protectors work too, but more against contusions and bruising than dislocations and the like. Nonetheless, they're not a bad investment to keep you—dermatologically anyway—in the pink.

Snowboarding

Many people believe that snowboarding is just like skiing, and that if you can do one, you can do the other. I can do the one (skiing) more than adequately. Imagine my surprise, therefore, when I finally tried the other (snowboarding) last year. As it turns out, I had a lot of company. Snowboarding is the world's fastest growing winter sport, and it's predicted that by the year 2000, there will be as many boarders as Alpine skiers.

In my case, the incentive was more personal. I had seen several of my friends leave for snowboarding vacations in previous winters and come back changed men. They wore their hair longer, no longer tucked in their shirts, and said "dude" and "tubular" a lot. Fancying myself a hep cat, I finally decided the time had come. I flew out West, rented the five-foot board, slung it over my shoulder, and asked the first guy I saw in trademark baggies the way to the slopes. Not long after, I finally stood at the summit, looking down at the pitches and moguls. With the hot knives of my skis, I knew that I could carve this kind of hill like a turkey. With the blunt shape of the board on the other hand . . . well, turkey was the word! I'd estimate I spent 30 percent of my time wobbling upright, and the other 70 percent flat on my back with snowmelt trickling down my inseam, doing my best to appear that I was professionally interested in cloud formations. The learning curve on a snowboard is so steep it's almost vertical, and the spills are like something out of a *Keystone Cop* movie. I never did find the inner Jack Kerouac that day, and as I trudged back to the lodge, bruised and aching, felt a phrase rise, unasked, to my lips. The phrase was the following: "I'm too old for this!"

Snowboarding Injuries Because you're not encumbered with two planks, as you are with skis, the chances of lower-extremity injuries while snowboarding are lessened significantly—they happen, but rarely. Major knee injuries like ACL tears occur with a frequency one quarter that of Alpine skiing accidents. But there are **ankle injuries** to beware of, and other problems, too. As you might expect, the wrist comes in for some serious abuse, from having to break all those falls! There is a plethora of other problems having to do with **shoulder dislocations** and **neck strains**. Because the board doesn't release like skis do, you do a lot of tumbling, head over heels.

Experts say that using soft-shelled boots as opposed to hard can cut down on injuries when you fall. But the best remedy for snowboarding accidents is a simple one: lessons. In a recent study of Swiss snowboarders, an impressive 80 percent of those surveyed traced their accident to riding mistakes and insufficient training. Because of the relative simplicity of the technique of snowboarding, most beginner students can advance to an intermediate level after their first lesson, and within a few days a novice can progress as far or further than a beginning skiier can in a couple of weeks. The moral of the story? Don't be like me, kids, stay in school!

Rock Climbing

Rock climbing is not an especially new sport, but it has never until recently, been anything that one could describe as a "boom sport." The alternative sports revolution has changed all that. There are now climbing centers, Alpine organizations, and "rock gyms" (gyms with climbing walls) in every fair-size city in the country, and climb-ins have become a kind of party event. For all ages and both sexes, this one-on-one challenge against the elements is showing signs of being a durably popular, quintessentially American sport.

Rock climbing has a range of approaches, from the technical—weighed down with ropes and safety devices—to the hairy extremes of free climbing, where you snake your way up a rockface based on simple arm and leg power, intuition, and guts. No matter how you cut it, rock climbing is a dance of strength and nerve. An experienced free-climber is a thing of beauty to watch as he or she grapples, shimmies, and seems sometimes nearly to sprint up a vertical wall. Strength, of course, is an essential element, and not just sheer muscle power, but conditioned strength, strength working in tandem with body knowledge. If you're simply strong, but don't know what you're doing, you can end up like the baseball pitcher with whom I was once climbing in the Grand Tetons. He put his arm out to get a handhold, tried to strong-arm himself up to the next pitch, and ended instead pulling his shoulder entirely out of joint in front of my horrified eyes. Though I snapped it back into place for him, he never pitched again.

Rock-Climbing Injuries The most common injuries to rock climbers, predictably enough, are to the hands. Four basic grips are used in rock climbing: open, cling, pocket, and pinch. But the physics involved isn't kind: when your entire body weight is hanging by the slender bones of the hands, those hands tend to suffer, as do the wrists and forearms. **Tendonitis, sprains, avulsion fractures, ligament strains**, and even **carpal tunnel syndrome** accrue to serious climbers. Taping the fingers, using thin rubber finger pads, and practicing range-of-motion exercises for the wrist and fingers can help prevent climbing injuries. The other injuries I won't talk about, because they mostly have to do with falling, and who wants to think about that? Instead, let's think about what you can do to climb injury-free.

Rock-climbing Tips

Stretching Particularly in rock climbing, where the body has to bear sudden weight on very concentrated parts of joints and limbs, stretching is one of the keys to prevent injuries. Specific areas to target if you're beginning to climb seriously are: **hamstring flexibility, hip flexibility, shoulder flexibility**, and **quadriceps flexibility**. On a related note, **never start climbing cold.** Do jumping jacks, jog in place—whatever it takes to get the blood flowing and the metabolism turning over.

Never Use Old Static Ropes If you're using a rope you probably know what you're doing anyway, but for you backyard dilettantes, it's important to remember: modern climbing ropes are high-tech items, which are what's called kernmantle-constructed (outer sheath over a high number of long internal filaments). The resulting construction allows them to stretch slightly, rather than snapping, and provides some extra shock protection at the end of any fall.

Know How to Tie Knots Knots are the key to safe technical climbing. Be sure before you go that you've got your overhand loop, bowline, figure-eight loop, and all the other party favorites down to a science.

Test Your Holds Loose rock is the enemy, but it's difficult to tell at a glance, so remember: strike all handholds with the heel of the hand before engaging them. Kick all footholds before setting your weight.

Finally, keep in mind that you should try to climb with some spring and rhythm. This is actually useful for conserving precious energy. Think flow, keep the breath moving—and don't look down!

Surfing

For those who haven't tried it: it's harder than it looks. For those who have, you know why you do it: because it's like nothing else. The famed Duke Kahanamouku, a wild and wiggy Hawaiian, brought it to the mainland around 1915, and it's been going strong ever since. Surfing actually dipped in popularity during the alternative sports revolution, and was brought back during the '90s in part by women, who began flocking to the freedom and to the unique mix of athletics and water joy that surfing provides. They were helped in this by the new, lighter, more-maneuverable twin-fin board, and a feeling among organizers of professional surfing contests that the sport needed a shot in the arm. Whatever the reason, women now represent a sizeable portion of the people out there braving the waves, and six women's surf shops have opened in Southern California in just the last year.

People who don't surf underestimate just how athletic surfing is. It requires flexibility, balance, and good upper and lower body strength. For those interested in getting into surfing seriously, experts generally recommend a conditioning program involving swimming, pushups (to better achieve that quick "pop-up" movement from lying down to standing up), crunches, and work on holding your breath (for those times when you're submerged under a wave).

Surfing Injuries

Typical injuries, as you might expect in a sport where you're spun and dropped from a great height, usually involved shoulder, back, and neck injuries. Another unpleasant side effect of all that cold-water immersion is Surfer's Ear. Known by the technical and unpleasant name of *exostosis*, it involves the ear bones actually beginning to grow again in reaction to all that uninsulated cold ocean pressing up against them. The result is a painful narrowing of the ear canal. And yet the remedy is simple: ear plugs.

That more sedate relative of surfing, windsurfing, generally causes its more enthusiastic practitioners to suffer from wrist and hand tendonitis (from gripping the boom to stay upright), and the occasional shoulder problems from being tossed violently into the drink.

Big-Wave Surfing

Lately showing signs of popularity among the adrenaline-deprived is big-wave surfing: that particular species of insanity that finds it fun to challenge a forty-foot high wall of moving water—a wall that weighs in the neighborhood of ten thousand tons! Three deaths in the mid '90s were attributed to big-wave surfing, but for the surfers and their fans, it provides a thrill like nothing else. Bigger waves obviously mean bigger wipeouts, and the drop off a forty-foot ledge of water can provide the neck-snapping fall to end all falls. But the biggest danger, according to veterans, is not the drop so much as the "hold-down," that minute or two in which you're kept pinned to the bottom by the churning water. Don't try this at home!

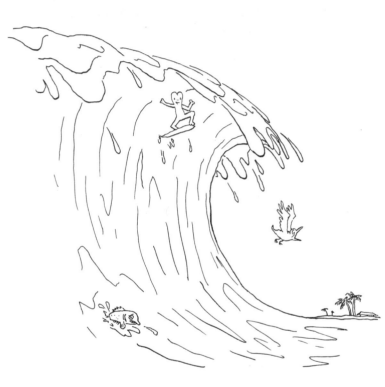

"Look, Ma, no brains!"

Skydiving

One could quite reasonably ask: why would a sensible human being, who lives in a nice house in the country, wears wingtip shoes and drives a station wagon, want to risk life and limb while being flushed from a plane like a frozen turd from the Boeing waste disposal unit? My friends tell me the rush of free fall is like nothing you can ever imagine—that's why, I suppose. Truth be told, it's next on my list. Two things to remember if you're a novice skydiver: your weight should be within the normal range (range for which the equipment was designated), and you should not have any respiratory problems—problems that can be aggravated by changes in altitude. Typical skydiving injuries I see have to do with botched landings: a high prevalence of **heel fractures, ankle sprains** and **fractures**, and **knee twists**. Those truly in need of thrills at all costs could check out skysurfing, which combines the zaniest elements of snowboarding and sky diving in one unholy package.

Epilogue

This page, alas, marks the end of our journey together. I've done my best to see that your time invested in this book was well spent. My goals were simple. I wanted to bring you the latest, most useful sports-medical information available, presented with an eye toward allowing you to heal quickly and perform athletically to the best of your abilities. I also wanted to permit you to diagnose your own injuries whenever possible, thereby saving you the time and expense of office visits. And last, I wanted to bring you into my own life as a doctor so that you never have to feel worried or alone in your discomfort. I know from my own experience that a little bedside manner goes a long way. And then there's sports. Where would I be without those thousands of hours of jogging, shooting hoops, skiing down virgin snowfields? Sports has provide me with some of the best company, the most stirring moments, and the deepest challenges of my life. I may love medicine, but sports will always be my first and truest love. So, as we say good-bye, I say to you, be of good health, stretch, be passionate, laugh as much as possible—and see you on the courts!

—ANDREW FELDMAN, M.D.

Appendix A

Med Units

• Note that when rehab exercises are prescribed, you should perform all of the exercises given for that part of the body. You should try to complete all of the reps and sets recommended for each exercise. However, if you feel you need to begin more slowly you should, by all means, work at your own pace. Turn to the corresponding rehab exercises in Appendix B (pages 176–192) for instructions on how to perform the rehab exercises prescribed.

• NSAI (Nonsteroidal Anti-inflammatory): These substances inhibit the inflammatory response of the body associated with injury and pain syndrome. They are not panacea but are intended as adjunctive treatment modalities. They can be purchased over the counter. An example of these are Nuprin, Advil, and Motrin. Your local chain drug store should also have generic brands. There are also scores of other available. Please be advised, as with any medicine, these do have side effects. Be sure to read the product information carefully before you use and follow proper dosage.

Shoulder

Instability

1. Rehab exercises.
2. Ice 2 times/day for 10–20 minutes for 2 weeks. Ice after sports or activity.
3. NSAI for 1–2 weeks.
4. Back to sports when pain-free (usually 6 weeks to 3 months).
5. Acute accidents should have X rays to rule out fracture.
6. If chronic instability becomes debilitating in sports or in life, surgery is indicated.

Redislocation or resubluxation occurs more often at a younger age and with frequency of activity.

Rotator Cuff Syndrome/Bursitis

1. Rehab exercises.
2. Ice 2 times/day for 10–20 minutes for 2 weeks. Ice after sports or activity.
3. NSAI for 1–2 weeks.
4. Avoid any activity that aggravates the injury until you are pain-free.
5. If pain persists for 3–4 months or worsens significantly, see a doctor. You may need to have an MRI or a cortisone shot.
6. If severe stiffness progresses (frozen shoulder), see a doctor immediately.

AC Joint Problems

1. Rehab exercises.
2. Ice 2 times/day for 10–20 minutes for 2 weeks. Ice after sports or activity.
3. NSAI for 1–2 weeks.
4. Resume sports as tolerated (usually after 4–6 weeks). Stretch before activity and ice after for 10–20 minutes.
5. If pain persists more than 3 months, see a doctor. You may need a cortisone shot or perhaps surgery.

Biceps Tendonitis

1. Any obvious physical deformity of the biceps should be seen by a doctor.
2. Rehab exercises.
3. Ice 2 times/day for 10–20 minutes for 2 weeks. Ice after sports or activity.
4. NSAI for 1–2 weeks.
5. Return to sports if pain-free (usually 2–4 weeks).
6. If pain persists for more than 8 weeks, see a doctor. Surgery is rarely necessary.

Muscular Aches and Pains of the Shoulder

1. Rehab exercises.
2. NSAI for 1–2 weeks.
3. Warm soaks in bathtub 2 times/day for 20 minutes.
4. Deep-tissue massage.
5. In cases of severe and chronic pain, postural training, an ergonomic chair, changes in your computer workstation, phone headset, acupuncture, or biofeedback may be necessary.
6. You may need to see a doctor at any time for a trigger-point injection of cortisone.

Hip, Thigh, and Groin

Quad, Groin (Adductor), Hamstring, Abductor Strains or Tears

1. Severity of disability = severity of strain.
2. Prevention is always the best cure. This includes stretching, strengthening, and balancing the strength of all the leg muscles, and proper form.
3. Ice 2 times/day for 10–20 minutes for 2 weeks. Ice after sports or activity.
4. NSAI for 1–2 weeks.
5. Rehab exercises.
6. Return to activity when tenderness subsides (usually 7–10 days for mild strains).

7. Severe strains can last up to 3–4 months. If pain persists see a doctor. Strains can become chronic and cause discomfort for many years.
8. Apply moist heat to the area before sports or activity to help warm up the large muscle. You can either soak in a warm bath or use a hydrocolator—a moist heating pad.
9. A large neoprene sleeve may help to give added support in activity until you are completely pain-free.

Hip Bursitis

1. Rehab exercises.
2. Ice 2 times/day for 10–20 minutes for 2 weeks. Ice after sports or activity.
3. NSAI for 1–2 weeks.
4. If pain persists for more than 6–8 weeks, see a doctor. You may need an injection of cortisone.

Elbow

Tennis Elbow (Lateral Epicondylitis)

1. Check equipment (racket and strings, balls). Ask a pro if necessary.
2. Check technique (grip, stroke, overall form). Ask a pro.
3. Rehab exercises.
4. Ice 2 times/day for 10–20 minutes for 2 weeks. Ice after sports or activity.
5. NSAI for 1–2 weeks.
6. Avoid activity that aggravates injury until you are pain-free.
7. Resume activity as tolerated. Tennis elbow can often take 2–6 months to heal.
8. A tennis elbow band may be helpful and acupuncture may work as well.
9. If pain persists past 2–3 months, see a doctor. You may need a cortisone shot or surgery.

Golfer's Elbow (Medial Epicondylitis)

1. Follow therapy for Tennis Elbow exactly. If you use an elbow band, place pads at inner elbow.

Bursitis

1. Rehab exercises.
2. Ice 2 times/day for 10–20 minutes, for 2 weeks. Ice after sports or activity.
3. NSAI for 1–2 weeks.
4. Bursitis is usually self-limiting. Return to activity as tolerated.
5. If elbow is severely reddened or painful, see a doctor. There is the danger of infection.
6. If bursitis is recurrent or painful, see a doctor. You may need to have the elbow surgically drained.

Biceps Tendonitis:

1. Ice 2 times/day for 10–20 minutes for 1–2 weeks. Ice after sports or activity.
2. NSAI for 1–2 weeks.
3. Rehab exercises.
4. Avoid curls or lifting with flex arms.
5. A neoprene elbow band may be helpful for sports and activity.
6. If pain persists for more than 6–8 weeks, see a doctor.

Hand and Wrist

Carpal Tunnel Syndrome

1. Rehab exercises.
2. Ice 2 times/day for 10–20 minutes for 2 weeks. Ice after sports, activity, and using the computer for an extended period of time.
3. NSAI for 1–2 weeks.
4. Symptoms come on gradually and are often self-limiting.
5. Wrist splints with rigid support will help. These are usually carried in orthopedic supply stores and can be custom-fitted.

6. Try to avoid activity that aggravates the injury. Modify your computer workstation, change the handlebar grips on your bike, and so forth.
7. If symptoms continue for 6–8 weeks with weakness or persistent numbness, see a doctor. You may need a cortisone shot or possible surgery to open up the carpal tunnel.

Ganglion/Cyst

1. Most times a ganglion is asymtomatic.
2. Most go away by themselves.
3. You can see a doctor for drainage or removal.

Mallet Finger

1. You'll need to see a doctor who will provide you with a custom splint. Most times this is not a problem that requires surgery.

Trigger Finger

1. Usually self-limiting.
2. NSAI for 1–2 weeks.
3. If pain persists or function is compromised see a doctor.

Wrist Tendonitis (de Quarvain's and Extensor Syndrome)

1. Ice 2 times/day for 10–20 minutes for 2 weeks. Ice after sports, activity, or using the computer for an extended period of time.
2. NSAI for 1–2 weeks.
3. Rehab exercises.
4. Return to full activity when pain-free.
5. An imobilizing brace may be helpful until pain is gone. You can find one at a surgical-supply store.
6. If pain persists for more than 1 or 2 months, see a doctor. You may need a cortisone injection or surgery.

Spine and Back

Low Back Strain

1. If you have pain, numbness, or tingling in your buttocks or down your leg, see a doctor.
2. Warm soaks 3 times/day (in bath or with a hydroculator).
3. Try to sleep on your side, in the fetal position. It may help to put a pillow between your knees.
4. Be sure to always bend at the knees and not from the waist when lifting anything, even a light object.
5. Rehab exercises.
6. NSAI for 1–2 weeks.
7. The use of a lumbar corset may help for sitting and driving.
8. If pain persists and does not improve within 2–4 weeks, see a doctor to check for a slipped disc.

Knee

Medial/Lateral Collateral Ligament Strain or Tear

1. Rehab exercises.
2. Ice 2 times/day for 10–20 minutes for 1–2 weeks. Ice after sports or activity.
3. NSAI for 1–2 weeks.
4. Healing is determined directly by the severity of the injury—anywhere from 6 weeks to 4 months.
5. Resume activity when comfortable doing so. You may need a neoprene brace with supports for sports.
6. It is wise to see a doctor if you have persistent, debilitating pain.

Meniscus Tear

1. Rehab exercises.
2. Ice 2 times/day for 10–20 minutes for 1–2 weeks. Ice after sports or activity.
3. NSAI for 1–2 weeks.
4. A neoprene brace may be necessary for sports.

5. If pain or locking of knee persists for more than 1–2 weeks, see a doctor. Surgery may be necessary.

Patella-Femoral Syndrome

1. Check for flat feet. You may need orthotics.
2. Rehab exercises.
3. Ice 2 times/day for 10–20 minutes for 2 weeks. Ice after sports or activity.
4. Avoid painful activity. Try cross-training for rest and relief.
5. A neoprene sleeve with a patellar cutout (donut) for sports may be helpful.
6. If pain persists for more than 3–6 months, see a doctor. Surgery is sometimes (although not often) necessary.

Iliotibial Band Tendonitis

1. Check for flat feet. You may need orthotics.
2. Check all of your athletic shoes for wear.
3. Rehab exercises.
4. Ice 2 times/day for 10–20 minutes. Ice after sports or activity.
5. NSAI for 1–2 weeks.
6. Cross-train to rest the injury and take the stress off your knee.
7. Run on soft surfaces. Avoid concrete and treadmills.
8. If problem persists for more than 4 weeks, see a doctor. Healing time can take up to 4–6 months. A cortisone shot may be necessary. Surgery is rare.

Patella Tendonitis

1. Check athletic shoes for wear.
2. Rehab exercises.
3. Ice 2 times/day for 10–20 minutes for 2 weeks. Ice after sports or activity.
4. NSAI for 1–2 weeks.
5. Cross-train to rest the injury and take stress of the knee.
6. A circumferential brand brace may be helpful. This is a constrictive band worn just below the kneecap.

7. Resume activity as tolerated. If pain persists for more than 2–3 months, see a doctor. Surgery is rarely recommended.

Shin Splints

1. Check athletic shoes for wear.
2. Check for flat feet. You may need orthotics.
3. Avoid hard running surfaces like concrete and treadmills.
4. Rehab exercises.
5. Ice 2 times/day for 10–20 minutes. Ice after sports or activity.
6. NSAI for 1–2 weeks.
7. Resume activity when there is no more pain. If pain persists for more than 4 weeks, see a doctor. There is the possibility of a stress fracture.

Foot

Turf Toe

1. Wear stiff-toed shoes, like a workboot if possible, for comfort.
2. Ice 2 times/day for 10–20 minutes. Ice after sports or activity.
3. NSAI for 1–2 weeks.
4. Symptoms should improve after 6 weeks. However, if injury inhibits sports or pain persists for long, see a doctor. A cortisone shot may be necessary or possible surgery.

Caused by repeated trauma to the joint in the big toe.

Metatarsalgia and Sesamoiditis

1. Rehab exercises.
2. Ice 2 times/day for 10–20 minutes for 2 weeks. Ice after sports or activity.
3. NSAI for 1–2 weeks.
4. Usually self-limiting. Resume activity as tolerated (usually after 1–6 weeks).
5. A soft foot pad or orthotic in front of the ball of the foot can be helpful.
6. If injury becomes chronic, see a doctor.

Plantar Fasciitis (Heel Spur)

1. Check athletic shoes for wear.
2. Check for flat feet. You may need orthotics.
3. Rehab exercises.
4. Ice 2 times/day for 10–20 minutes for 1–2 weeks. Ice after sports or activity.
5. NSAI for 1–2 weeks.
6. Placing a heel cup or gel pad in all of your shoes may be helpful.
7. If pain persists for more than 8–12 weeks, see a doctor.

Morton's Neuroma

1. Ice 2 times/day for 10–20 minutes for 2 weeks. Ice after sports or activity.
2. NSAI for 1–2 weeks.
3. Wear shoes with a wide toe box.
4. Cotton pads between the toes or a soft pad under the foot can also be helpful.
5. If pain persists for more than 8–12 weeks, see a doctor. If symptoms are unremitting after 6–8 months, surgery may be necessary.

Due to tight shoes or overuse.

Tendonitis of the Foot

1. Check athletic shoes for wear.
2. Check for flat feet. You may need orthotics.
3. Ice 2 times/day for 10–20 minutes for 2 weeks. Ice after sports or activity.
4. NSAI for 1–2 weeks.
5. Cross-train and decrease activity.
6. Rehab exercises when pain-free.
7. A soft pad applied to the area when wearing shoes may be helpful.
8. If pain persists for more than 6 weeks, see a doctor.

Bunion

1. Try to wear wide shoes for greater comfort. Go barefoot at home whenever possible.
2. If pain is persistent or if there is a severe cosmetic deformity, surgery may be necessary.

Ankle

Sprains of the Ankle

1. Healing time = the severity of the sprain.
2. Any pain but the most minor should be seen by a doctor and treated with an X ray in case of fracture.
3. Ice 2 times/day for 10–20 minutes for 2 weeks. Ice after sports or activity.
4. NSAI for 1–2 weeks.
5. Elevate the ankle whenever possible. This will help to reduce swelling.
6. A sprain may take 3 weeks to 4 months to heal.
7. Return to activity when you are almost pain-free with almost complete strength back. Cross-train until then with sports that won't aggravate the injury.
8. A support brace may be necessary for approximately 4 weeks after you return to activity. An orthopedic supply store will have a brace custom-fitted.

Achilles Tendonitis/Rupture

1. Check athletic shoes for wear.
2. Check for flat feet. You may need orthotics.
3. Rehab exercises.
4. Ice 2 times/day for 10–20 minutes for 2 weeks. Ice after sports or activity.
5. Return to activity when pain-free. Cross-train until then with sports that won't aggravate the injury.
6. A heel lift in all of your shoes may be helpful. Higher-heeled shoes—not too high!—(a workboot or cowboy boot for men) may also help alleviate discomfort.
7. If pain persists for more than 8 weeks, see a doctor.

Appendix B

Rehab Exercises and Stretches

- Note that all exercises and stretches are performed at a standard of 10 repetitions, 3 times per day. If, at first, the number of repetitions is too difficult, you should either limit the repetitions or decrease the amount of weight you are using for the exercise. However, you should strive for the prescribed number of reps.

- If the reps are too easy for you, you should increase the weight (or the tension if you are using an elastic band). A general rule of thumb is that the first 5 reps should be easy, reps 6–8 should be difficult, and reps 9–10 should be shy of a struggle. This rule should help you determine if you are using an appropriate weight. It's good to start with a 2-pound weight and progress from there.

- Exercises should be "held" for a few seconds. Stretches should be "held" for between 15 and 30 seconds. Be sure not to bounce when you stretch. Rather hold and increase the stretch in a smooth steady motion without pulling or straining.

- Weights, cuff weights, and rubber tubing (or elastic bands) can be purchased at a sporting-goods store or a medical-supply store.

SHOULDER EXERCISES

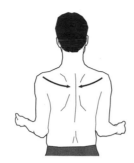

1. Stand with elbows bent to 90 degrees.
2. Pinch shoulder blades together as you rotate arms outward.
3. Hold.
4. 10 repetitions, 3 times per day.

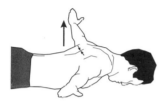

1. Lie on belly with arms at 90 degrees out to side.
2. Pinch shoulder blades together as shown.
3. Raise arms a few inches off floor.
4. Hold and slowly lower.
5. 10 repetitions, 3 times per day.

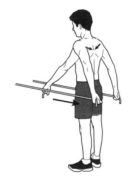

1. Anchor rubber tubing to a solid object.
2. Stand holding rubber tubing in both hands with arms in front of body.
3. Pinch shoulder blades backward as shown.
4. Holding the shoulder blades stable, pull arms backward.
5. Hold, then slowly relax.
6. 10 repetitions, 3 times per day.

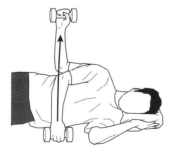

1. Hold weight in your hand.
2. Lie on side so that arm holding weight is on top.
3. Rotate arm upward, keeping elbow bent as shown.
4. Hold, then slowly lower.
5. 10 repetitions, 3 times per day for each shoulder.

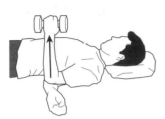

1. Hold weight in your hand.
2. Lie on back with elbow bent, forearm parallel with floor.
3. Rotate arm in toward body, keeping elbow bent as shown.
4. Hold, then slowly lower.
5. 10 repetitions, 3 times per day for each shoulder.

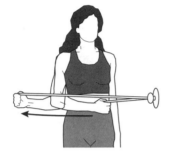

1. Anchor rubber tubing to a solid object.
2. Grasp rubber tubing in hand as shown.
3. Rotate arm outward, keeping elbow bent and close to the body.
4. Hold, then slowly lower.
5. 10 repetitions, 3 times per day for each shoulder.

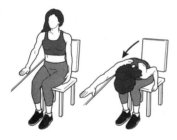

SHOULDER STRETCHES

1. Sit in a chair with arm on table as shown.
2. Bend forward in the chair, sliding the arm forward on the table, so that you feel a stretch.
3. Hold.
4. 10 repetitions, 3 times per day for each shoulder.

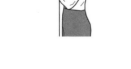

1. Stand near a wall as shown.
2. Slowly "walk" your fingers up the wall, so that you feel a stretch.
3. Hold.
4. 10 repetitions, 3 times per day for each shoulder.

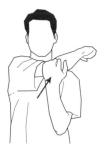

1. Stand grasping elbow with other hand as shown.
2. Pull the elbow and arm across your chest so that you feel a stretch.
3. Hold.
4. 10 repetitions, 3 times per day for each shoulder.

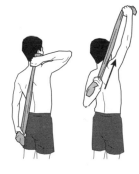

1. Stand in doorway with elbows bent and hands placed on door frame as shown.
2. Lean your body forward so that you feel a stretch.
3. Hold.
4. 10 repetitions, 3 times per day.

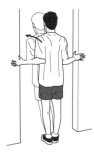

1. Stand with towel or cane as shown, arm behind your back.
2. Stretch the arm up behind your back by pulling upward on the towel with the other hand for assistance.
3. Hold.
4. 10 repetitions, 3 times per day for each shoulder.

HIP, THIGH, AND GROIN EXERCISES

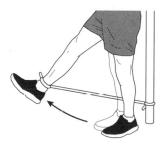

1. Anchor rubber tubing to solid object and ankle.
2. Pull leg forward as shown.
3. Hold, then slowly relax.
4. 10 repetitions, 3 times per day for each leg.

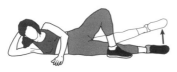

1. Place cuff weight around ankle.
2. Lie on side as shown, with leg on bottom.
3. Raise leg up toward ceiling.
4. Hold, then slowly relax.
5. 10 repetitions, 3 times per day for each leg.

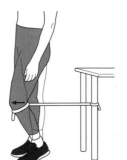

1. Anchor rubber tubing to solid object and ankle as shown.
2. Stand with toe pointed out to side.
3. Now cross the leg in front of your other leg.
4. Hold, then slowly relax.
5. 10 repetitions, 3 times per day for each leg.

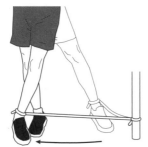

1. Arrange tubing around leg as shown.
2. Begin with knee straight, then slowly bend knee partway (about one-third).
3. Slowly straighten knee again.
4. 10 repetitions, 3 times per day for each leg.

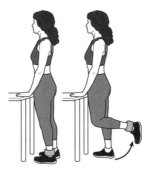

1. Stand holding onto solid object as shown.
2. Place weight on ankle.
3. Slowly bend knee to almost a 90 degree angle.
4. Hold, then slowly lower.
5. 10 repetitions, 3 times per day for each leg.

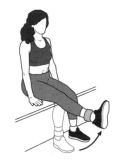

1. Sit on edge of table or bed.
2. Place weight around foot.
3. Straighten knee and stop approx. 30 degrees from full extension.
4. Hold, then slowly lower.
5. 10 repetitions, 3 times per day for each leg.

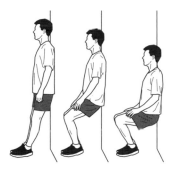

1. Stand with back against wall, feet shoulder-width apart and 18 inches from wall.
2. Slowly slide down wall halfway. Squeeze ball or pillow between knees.
3. Hold.
4. 10 repetitions, 3 times per day.

HIP, THIGH, AND GROIN STRETCHES

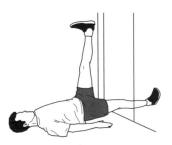

1. Lie on back with leg propped in doorway as shown.
2. Keep the opposite leg straight on the floor.
3. Lie as close to the base of the doorway as possible while keeping the leg straight.
4. Hold.
5. 10 repetitions, 3 times per day for each leg.

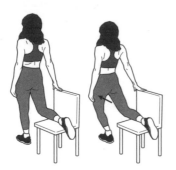

1. Assume position shown, with knee on chair.
2. Bend the opposite knee so that you feel a stretch.
3. Do not allow your lower back to arch.
4. Hold.
5. 10 repetitions, 3 times per day for each leg.

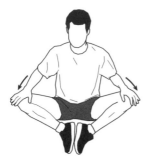

1. Sit with knees bent, feet together as shown.
2. Press knees downward toward the floor, using hands as needed.
3. Hold.
4. 10 repetitions, 3 times per day.

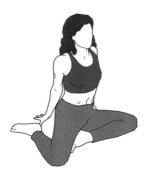

1. Sit with your right leg bent and your right heel just outside of your right hip.
2. Bend your left leg and place the sole of your left foot next to the inside of your upper right leg. Place your hands on the floor behind you to support your upper body.
3. Hold.
4. 10 repetitions, 3 times per day for each leg.

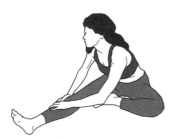

1. Straighten your right leg with the knee slightly bent; move the sole of your left foot until it is just touching the inside of your right thigh.
2. Slowly bend forward from your hips to create the feeling of an easy stretch in the hamstrings.
3. Hold.
4. 10 repetitions, 3 times per day for each leg.

ELBOW EXERCISES

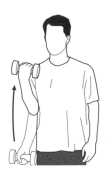

1. Stand with arm straight, palm facing forward as shown.
2. Hold dumbbell weight.
3. Bend elbow as shown.
4. Hold.
5. 10 repetitions, 3 times per day for each elbow.

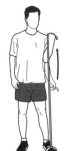

1. Stand holding elastic tubing with hand and the other tied to foot as shown.
2. Keep palm facing forward as shown.
3. Bend elbow as shown.
4. Hold, then slowly lower.
5. 10 repetitions, 3 times per day for each elbow.

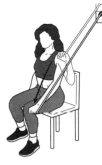

1. Anchor the elastic tubing to something solid.
2. Sit in a chair and hold elastic tubing in hand with elbow bent as shown.
3. Push hand down to straighten elbow.
4. Hold, then slowly relax.
5. 10 repetitions, 3 times per day for each elbow.

ELBOW STRETCHES

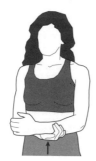

1. Bend elbow as shown, as much as you can.
2. Try to bend it further with the other hand until you feel a stretch.
3. Hold.
4. 10 repetitions, 3 times per day for each elbow.

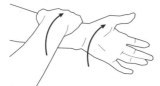

1. Turn palm of hand upward as shown.
2. Use the other hand on wrist to help so that you feel a stretch.
3. Hold.
4. 10 repetitions, 3 times per day for each elbow.

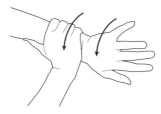

1. Turn palm of hand downward as shown.
2. Use other hand on wrist to help so that you feel a stretch.
3. Hold.
4. 10 repetitions, 3 times per day for each elbow.

HAND AND WRIST EXERCISES

1. Sit or stand with arm supported as shown.
2. Hold weight in hand.
3. Curl wrist slowly upward.
4. Hold, then, slowly lower.
5. 10 repetitions, 3 times per day for each hand.

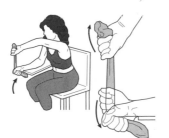

1. Sit or stand with arm supported as shown.
2. Hold the loose end of the elastic tubing with your other hand to apply resistance.
3. Curl wrist slowly upward.
4. Hold, then slowly lower.
5. 10 repetitions, 3 times per day for each hand.

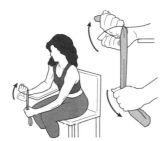

1. Sit or stand with arm supported as shown.
2. Hold loose end of the elastic tubing with your other hand to apply resistance.
3. Bend wrist downward as show.
4. Hold, then slowly return to start position.
5. 10 repetitions, 3 times per day for each hand.

WRIST STRETCHES

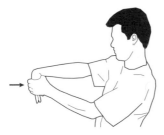

1. Hold wrist as shown.
2. Bend the wrist until you feel a stretch.
3. Hold.
4. 10 repetitions, 3 times per day for each wrist.

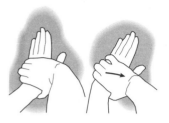

1. Place wrist flat on table as shown.
2. Use the other hand to bend the wrist inward (toward thumb) until you feel a stretch.
3. Hold.
4. 10 repetitions, 3 times per day for each wrist.

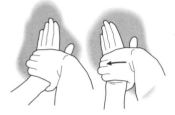

1. Place wrist flat on table as shown.
2. Use the other hand to bend the wrist outward (toward little finger) until you feel a stretch.
3. Hold.
4. 10 repetitions, 3 times per day for each wrist.

BACK AND SPINE EXERCISES

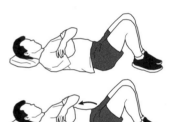

1. Lie on back with knees bent.
2. Tighten abdominal muscles, squeeze buttock muscles, and flatten back into the floor as shown.
3. Hold.
4. 10 repetitions, 3 times per day.

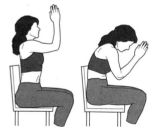

1. Sit in a straight-backed chair.
2. Tighten abdominal muscles, squeeze buttock muscles, and flatten your back against chair as shown.
3. Hold.
4. 10 repetitions, 3 times per day.

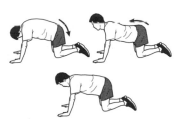

1. Assume hands and knees position.
2. Tighten abdominal muscles, squeeze buttock muscles, and tuck tailbone under, to hunch back upward as shown.
3. Then, slowly let lower back sag toward floor as you rotate tailbone upward to arch as shown.
4. Now, find your neutral (balanced) position.
5. Hold.
6. 10 repetitions, 3 times per day.

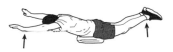

1. Lie on back with knees bent.
2. Cross arms over chest. Perform pelvic tilt and hold.
3. Raise head and shoulders just an inch off the floor, curl trunk upward as shown.
4. Hold.
5. 10 repetitions, 3 times per day.

---

1. Lie on belly over pillow, with arms overhead as shown.
2. Raise head, arms, and legs off floor as shown.
3. Hold.
4. 10 repetitions, 3 times per day.

BACK AND SPINE STRETCHES

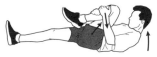

1. Lie on back.
2. Pull knee to chest.
3. Hold.
4. 10 repetitions, 3 times per day for each knee.

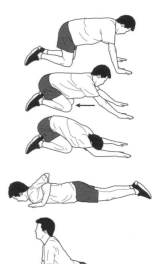

1. Assume hands and knees position.
2. Bend knees to move buttocks toward heels as shown.
3. Hold.
4. 10 repetitions, 3 times per day.

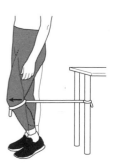

1. Assume position shown.
2. Straighten arms to press trunk upward, letting hips sag toward floor.
3. Hold.
4. 10 repetitions, 3 times per day.

KNEES EXERCISES

1. Arrange tubing around leg as shown.
2. Begin with knee straight, then slowly bend knee partway (about one-third).
3. Slowly straighten knee again.
4. 10 repetitions, 3 times per day for each knee.

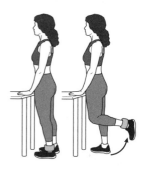

1. Stand holding onto solid object as shown.
2. Place weight on ankle.
3. Slowly bend knee to almost a 90 degree angle.
4. Hold, then slowly lower.
5. 10 repetitions, 3 times per day for each knee.

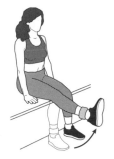

1. Sit on edge of table or bed.
2. Place weight around foot.
3. Straighten knee and stop approx. 30 degrees from full extension.
4. Hold, then slowly lower.
5. 10 repetitions, 3 times per day for each knee.

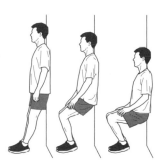

1. Stand with back against wall, feet shoulder-width apart and 18 inches from wall
2. Slowly slide down wall halfway. Squeeze ball or pillow between knees.
3. Hold.
4. 10 repetitions, 3 times per day.

KNEE STRETCHES

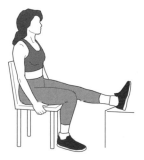

1. Sit with leg propped as shown.
2. Relax, letting the leg straighten.
3. Hold.
4. 10 repetitions, 3 times per day for each knee.

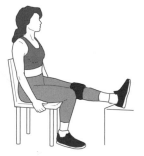

1. Place weight around knee.
2. Sit with leg propped as shown.
3. Relax, letting the leg straighten.
4. Hold.
5. 10 repetitions, 3 times per day for each knee.

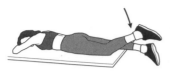

1. Lie on a table or bed with feet hanging over end as shown.
2. Slowly allow gravity to extend the knee.
3. Hold.
4. 10 repetitions, 3 times per day for each knee.

ANKLE EXERCISES

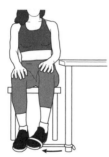

1. Place elastic tubing around foot as shown.
2. Push toes slowly away from your body.
3. Hold.
4. 10 repetitions, 3 times per day for each ankle.

---

1. Place elastic tubing around foot as shown.
2. Without moving your hip or knee, turn the bottom of your foot inward toward your body.
3. Hold.
4. 10 repetitions, 3 times per day for each ankle.

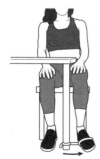

1. Place elastic tubing around your foot as shown.
2. Without moving your hip or knee, tip the bottom of your foot outward away from your body.
3. Hold.
4. 10 repetitions, 3 times per day for each ankle.

ANKLE STRETCHES

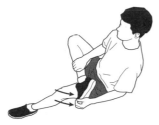

1. Assume position shown, pulling the toes toward your body so that you feel a stretch.
2. Hold.
3. 10 repetitions, 3 times per day for each ankle.

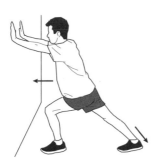

1. Position your body against a wall as shown with foot behind.
2. Point toes directly toward wall and hold heel down.
3. Lean into wall as shown so that you feel a stretch.
4. Hold.
5. 10 repetitions, 3 times per day for each ankle.

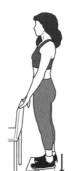

1. Place the front of your feet on a book or block, leaving your heels off the ground.
2. The book/block should be a few inches tall.
3. Hold onto a solid object standing upright as shown so that you feel a stretch.
4. Hold.
5. 10 repetitions, 3 times per day for each ankle.

FOOT EXERCISES

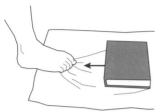

1. Sitting in a chair, place a towel flat on the floor in front of you.
2. Place your heel firmly on floor, forefoot on end of towel.
3. Without lifting your heel from the floor, use your toes to pull the towel toward you.
4. 5–10 repetitions 3 times per day.
5. To increase resistance, place a book on the end of the towel.

FOOT STRETCHES

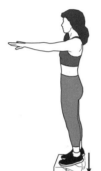

1. Stand on a step with heels hanging off the back edge, hands out in front of you.
2. Raise your heels as far as possible, then lower them as far as you can.
3. 10 repetitions, 3 times per day.

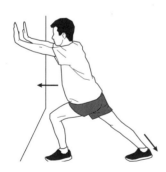

1. Position your body against a wall as shown with foot behind.
2. Point toes directly toward wall and hold heel down.
3. Lean into wall as shown so that you feel a stretch.
4. Hold.
5. 10 repetitions, 3 times per day.

INDEX

page numbers in **bold face** indicate illustrations